WALL PILATES WORKOUTS FOR WOMEN

EVERYTHING YOU NEED TO KNOW TO HAVE A PERFECT BODY

Winona Kenneth

WALL PILATES WORKOUTS FOR WOMEN: EVERYTHING YOU NEED TO KNOW TO HAVE A PERFECT BODY

Written by Winona Kenneth

First Edition

Copyrights Notice

Limited Liability

Please note that the content of this book is based on personal experience and various information sources.

Although the author has made every effort to present accurate, up-to-date, reliable, and complete information in this book, they make no representations or warranties concerning the accuracy or completeness of the content of this book and specifically disclaim any implied warranties of merchantability or fitness for a particular purpose.

Your particular circumstances may not be suited to the example illustrated in this book; in fact, they likely will not be. You should use the information in this book at your own risk.

All trademarks, service marks, product names, and the characteristics of any names mentioned in this book are considered the property of their respective owners and are used only for reference. No endorsement is implied when we use one of these terms.

This book is only for personal use. Please note the information contained within this document is for educational and entertainment purposes only and no warranties of any kind are declared or implied. Readers acknowledge that the author is not engaging in the rendering of legal, financial, or professional advice.

Please consult a licensed professional before attempting any techniques outlined in this book. Nothing in this book is intended to replace common sense legal accounting, or professional advice and is meant only to inform. By reading this document, the reader agrees that under no circumstances is the author responsible for any losses, direct or indirect, which are incurred as a result of the use of the information contained within this document, including, but not limited to, errors, omissions, or inaccuracies.

Table of Contents

Introduction

Welcome to the fascinating and beneficial world of Wall Pilates! This book has been created to guide you through a series of workouts specifically designed for women who wish to experience the many advantages of this innovative and accessible form of exercise.

Wall Pilates represents an evolution of traditional Pilates practices, offering a variety of targeted exercises that leverage the support of the wall to enhance strength, flexibility, and posture. With a careful approach to the fundamental principles of Pilates, this form of training provides a unique path to achieve your fitness goals effectively and in a balanced manner.

Throughout this book, we will explore the fundamentals of Pilates, learn basic and advanced exercises to be performed using the wall as an ally, and address specific topics such as muscle toning, weight management, and back issue prevention. Additionally, we will examine how to integrate Wall Pilates into your daily routine to maximize long-term benefits.

Whether you are a beginner or an experienced Pilates practitioner, this book is designed to be a comprehensive and inspiring resource, providing you with the knowledge and tools necessary to incorporate Wall Pilates into your life healthily and sustainably.

Prepare for an exciting journey toward physical and mental well-being through Wall Pilates. We are thrilled to share this experience with you and accompany you on the path to achieving your health and fitness goals. Happy training!

CHAPTER 1: PILATES FUNDAMENTALS: BASIC PRINCIPLES

The fundamental principles of Pilates form the cornerstone upon which this discipline is built and are crucial for a comprehensive understanding of how to perform exercises effectively. These principles provide the necessary guidance to extract the maximum benefits from Pilates, whether you are a beginner or an experienced practitioner. Let's delve into each principle in detail:

1-Control: Pilates emphasizes precise control of movements. Each exercise requires awareness and coordination to maintain muscular control throughout the range of motion.

2-Center (Powerhouse): This principle refers to the area of the body known as the "powerhouse" or "core," which includes the abdominal muscles, back muscles, glutes, and pelvic muscles. All Pilates exercises are designed to engage and strengthen the core.

3-Flow of Movement: Pilates encourages a smooth flow of movements without abrupt or excessive efforts. This principle aims to develop fluidity in movements, enhancing the mind-body connection.

4-Precision: Every movement in Pilates is targeted and intentional. Attention to precision ensures that each exercise is performed correctly to maximize benefits and reduce the risk of injury.

5-Breathing: Proper breathing is fundamental in Pilates. Controlled, full breaths are encouraged, and seamlessly integrated with movements, supporting the effectiveness of exercises and contributing to relaxation.

6-Concentration: Pilates demands mental concentration. Each exercise requires the individual's full attention to reap maximum benefits. Focusing on movement and the mind-body connection is essential.

7-Isolation of Movement: Pilates exercises often involve targeted work on specific muscle groups without excessive involvement of others. This allows for more focused and effective work on specific areas of the body.

Understanding and applying these basic principles are crucial to fully harness the potential of Pilates, establishing a solid foundation for ongoing practice and lasting benefits.

Control

The principle of "Control" in Pilates is fundamental and refers to the precision and conscious management of movements during the execution of exercises. This concept goes beyond the mere mechanical execution of exercises; it implies attentive awareness and mental engagement in every phase of movement.

Precise Movements. In Pilates, each movement is targeted to work on specific muscle groups. The practitioner must focus on precise execution, avoiding abrupt or uncontrolled movements.

Body Awareness. Control requires continuous awareness of one's own body during exercise. This involves a mind-body connection, where the practitioner is aware of how each part of the body moves and works.

Stability and Endurance. Control extends to stabilizing the body during movement. Maintaining stability requires constant muscular engagement, contributing to the development of strength and endurance.

Injury Prevention. Accurate control reduces the risk of injuries. By avoiding excessively fast or uncoordinated movements, joints are protected, and proper form is promoted.

Respiratory Integration. Control also extends to managing breathing. Proper breathing is integrated with movements to support stability and precise execution.

Maintaining control during the execution of Pilates exercises is crucial to maximize benefits and improve the connection between mind and body. This principle translates into a more mindful practice, promotes proper muscle development, and contributes to the overall well-being of the practitioner in the long term

Center (POWERHOUSE)

The principle of the "Powerhouse" in Pilates is essential and refers to the area of the body also known as the "powerhouse." This region includes the muscles of the abdomen, back, glutes, and pelvic muscles. The conscious activation and strengthening of this area are crucial to ensure stability and strength during the execution of exercises.

Engagement of Core Muscles. Pilates places particular emphasis on the active engagement of the muscles in the "Powerhouse." These muscles work together to provide the necessary stability to perform exercises effectively.

Support for the Spine. Strengthening the "Powerhouse" contributes to supporting the spine, reducing the risk of strains or injuries to the back. This is essential for maintaining proper posture and preventing muscle and joint issues.

Power Generation. The strength from the "Powerhouse" acts as a central point for power generation during many Pilates exercises. This area is the focal point from which the necessary force is developed for other body movements.

Movement Control. A well-trained "Powerhouse" provides the foundation for precise control of movements. It helps avoid uncontrolled movements and promotes a smooth and coordinated flow.

Mind-Body Connection. Attention to the "Powerhouse" fosters the mind-body connection. By focusing on this area, the practitioner develops greater awareness of their body during exercise.

Adaptability to Skill Levels. The concept of the "Powerhouse" is adaptable to different skill levels. Whether for beginners or experienced individuals, working in this area allows for gradual and continuous progress in muscle strengthening.

Maintaining a strong and active "Powerhouse" is a key pillar of Pilates, essential for achieving lasting benefits, improving overall body strength, and promoting optimal muscle and postural health.

Flow of Movement

The principle of "Flow of Movement" in Pilates emphasizes the importance of executing exercises with a smooth and continuous motion, avoiding excessive effort or abrupt movements. This concept is based on the philosophy that uninterrupted and controlled movement not only enhances the mind-body connection but also maximizes physical benefits.

Continuity in Movements. In Pilates, the goal is to create a sequence of movements that flow seamlessly from one to the next. This requires constant commitment and effortless transition between different phases of the exercises.

Mind-Body Connection. The flow of movement promotes a deeper connection between the mind and body. Maintaining constant awareness of movements and breathing creates a more engaging experience during the workout.

Coordination and Control. Smooth movement requires precise coordination and careful control. This principle encourages the practitioner to perform exercises with precision, ensuring that each part of the body moves in harmony with the others.

Reducing Joint Stress. Controlled flow contributes to reducing stress on the joints. By avoiding abrupt movements, joints are protected from potential injuries, promoting greater safety during exercise.

Improving Endurance. The continuous and controlled execution of exercises contributes to improving muscle endurance. This type of training aims to gradually build strength without excessively fatiguing the muscles.

Harmonious Experience. The ultimate goal of the flow of movement is to create a harmonious experience during the workout. This not only makes exercises more effective but can also make the entire training process more enjoyable and rewarding.

Integrating the principle of the flow of movement into Pilates practice helps make exercises more efficient, promotes greater body awareness, and contributes to better movement quality in the long run.

Precision

The principle of "Precision" in Pilates emphasizes the importance of performing each movement and exercise with the utmost accuracy and attention to detail. This concept is crucial to ensure that exercises are executed correctly, maximizing benefits, and reducing the risk of injuries. Let's delve into what the Precision principle entails in the context of Pilates:

Control in Movements. Precision requires accurate control at every phase of movement. This means avoiding disjointed or sloppy movements and maintaining a conscious and targeted management of each action.

Body Alignment. Pilates exercises emphasize correct body alignment. Maintaining proper posture during exercises is essential to optimally engage target muscles and prevent excessive stress on joints and muscles.

Specific Muscle Engagement. Every Pilates exercise aims to involve specific muscle groups. Precision involves the targeted engagement of these muscles without overloading them and without excessively involving other muscle groups.

Coordinated Breathing. Precision extends to coordinating breathing with movements. Maintaining controlled and coordinated breathing helps support stability and movement precision.

Adaptation to Skill Level. The concept of precision is adaptable to different skill levels. Whether you are a beginner learning the basics or an advanced practitioner refining more complex exercises, precision is always crucial.

Constant Awareness. Precision requires constant awareness of what the body is doing at every moment. This mindful attention contributes to improving the mind-body connection and optimizing results.

Maintaining precision in the execution of Pilates exercises is essential to fully harness the benefits of this discipline. Conscious attention to detail contributes to creating a more effective, safe, and rewarding Pilates practice in the long run.

Breathing

The principle of "Breathing" in Pilates emphasizes the importance of controlled, coordinated, and mindful breathing during the execution of exercises. Proper breathing is a fundamental element in Pilates, contributing both to supporting movement and maintaining an effective mind-body connection. Let's delve into what the Breathing principle entails in the context of Pilates:

Lateral Breathing. In Pilates, lateral breathing is often encouraged, meaning the expansion of the ribs during inhalation. This type of breathing allows for a fuller engagement of respiratory muscles, promoting trunk stabilization.

Involvement of the Diaphragm. Correct breathing involves the diaphragm, the main muscle of respiration. Consciously inhaling and exhaling promotes complete ventilation and activation of the "core."

Coordination with Movements. Breathing in Pilates is coordinated with movements. Typically, inhalation occurs before the movement, preparing the body, while exhalation accompanies the movement itself, facilitating control and precision.

Stabilization of the "Powerhouse". Proper breathing contributes to the stabilization of the "Powerhouse," the central area of the body. This stabilization is crucial for performing exercises with control and strength.

Tension Reduction. Awareness of breathing helps reduce tension. Regular and controlled breathing can promote muscle relaxation and contribute to increased body awareness.

Mind-Body Connection. Breathing in Pilates is an integral part of the mind-body connection. Focusing on breathing allows the practitioner to be more aware of their body, enhancing attention and concentration during exercises.

Integrating correct breathing into Pilates movements is essential to maximize the benefits of training. Mindful breathing contributes not only to physically supporting exercises but also to creating a more centered, relaxed, and effective experience within the context of Pilates practice.

Concentration

The principle of "Concentration" in Pilates emphasizes the importance of maintaining precise and mindful mental focus during the execution of exercises. Concentration in Pilates goes beyond mere mechanical execution, involving the mind in every aspect of movement to maximize benefits and improve the mind-body connection. Let's delve into what the Concentration principle entails in the context of Pilates:

Focus on Every Movement. Concentration requires full attention to every executed movement. This means being aware of how the body moves, muscle sensations, and nuances of the movement to ensure accurate execution.

Present Mind. Concentration in Pilates requires being completely present during the workout. Eliminating external distractions and focusing on the execution of the exercise helps maximize benefits and avoid errors due to lack of attention.

Correction of Postural Habits. Mental awareness enables the correction of incorrect postural habits. Being concentrated during exercises helps identify and correct any postural imbalances, improving overall posture.

Improvement of Precision. Concentration is essential for improving precision in movements. Keeping the mind focused on correct execution helps avoid disjointed movements and promotes more accurate control.

Integration with Breathing. Concentration integrates with breathing, ensuring that each movement is coordinated with the breathing rhythm. This synchronicity contributes to a harmonious flow during exercises.

Development of Mind-Body Connection. Concentration fosters the development of the mind-body connection. When the mind is fully engaged in the execution of exercises, a synergy between the mind and body is created, enhancing the effectiveness of the workout.

Maintaining concentration during Pilates practice is crucial for optimal results. Focused mindfulness contributes not only to the correct execution of exercises but also to increased body awareness and a deeper connection between the mind and movement.

Isolation of Movement

The principle of "Isolation of Movement" in Pilates emphasizes the ability to perform exercises by focusing on specific muscle groups without excessively involving others. This concept is crucial for working precisely on certain areas of the body and for developing strength and flexibility more accurately. Let's delve into what the Isolation of Movement principle entails in the context of Pilates:

Focus on Specific Muscle Groups. During exercises, attention is directed to specific muscle groups. The goal is to isolate these muscle groups, allowing them to play a predominant role in the execution of the exercise.

Minimization of the Influence of Other Muscles. During the isolation of movement, efforts are made to minimize the influence of other muscles not involved in the exercise. This allows focusing effort and attention on a specific area, promoting more targeted muscle development.

Precision in Execution. Isolation of movement requires precision in the execution of exercises. By focusing on a single muscle group, the practitioner can refine form and improve the quality of movement.

Development of Strength and Flexibility. Focusing on individual muscle groups allows for more targeted development of strength and flexibility. This is particularly beneficial for those looking to improve specific aspects of their physical fitness.

Prevention of Muscle Imbalances. Isolation of movement helps prevent muscle imbalances. Working on specific muscle groups contributes to maintaining balance in overall muscle strength.

Adaptability to Different Levels. The concept of isolation of movement can be adapted to different skill levels. Both beginners and experts can benefit from isolation exercises, adjusting resistance and complexity based on their abilities.

Isolation of Movement in Pilates allows for personalized training, refining, and strengthening of specific muscle groups to enhance overall strength, flexibility, and physical fitness.

CHAPTER 2: PREPARATION AND NECESSARY EQUIPMENT

Introduction to the Chapter: Preparation and Necessary Equipment

Welcome to the chapter dedicated to "Preparation and Necessary Equipment" for your wall-based Pilates training journey. The key to a rewarding and effective Pilates experience lies in proper preparation and the appropriate use of equipment. In this chapter, we will explore in detail how to set up your training space, select the right tools, and prepare your body to reap the maximum benefits from each wall Pilates session.

Correctly preparing the training environment is crucial to ensure a safe, comfortable, and stimulating space. We will discuss the essential elements to consider in creating your workout area, from choosing the ideal location to organizing equipment to maximize the efficiency of exercises.

Beyond the physical preparation of the training environment, we will also delve into the importance of selecting the right equipment for wall Pilates practice. From choosing mats and straps to resistance bands and other specific tools, we will guide you in creating a well-equipped "Pilates home."

Additionally, we will explore warm-up exercises that can help prepare the body, improve flexibility, and ready the muscles for more intense workouts. Body preparation is a key element in maximizing the benefits of every Pilates session, and we will provide you with a series of targeted exercises to optimize your performance.

Are you ready to dive into creating a supportive training environment and discovering the equipment that will make your wall Pilates journey a rewarding experience? Keep reading to gain the fundamental knowledge to prepare your mind and body to make the most of each Pilates session.

Preparation and Necessary Equipment

The chapter "Preparation and Necessary Equipment" focuses on two crucial aspects of a successful training experience in the context of Wall Pilates. Let's delve into what this chapter entails:

Preparation: This section of the chapter deals with how to prepare the training environment to maximize the effectiveness of Wall Pilates exercises. This includes choosing the ideal location, organizing the space, and creating a safe and comfortable environment. The physical preparation of the environment plays a fundamental role in fostering consistent and distraction-free practice, allowing the practitioner to fully focus on the exercises.

Necessary Equipment: This part of the chapter addresses the selection and proper use of equipment for Wall Pilates. It includes choosing mats, straps, resistance bands, and other specific tools needed to perform exercises effectively. The section provides detailed information on how to use these tools safely, illustrating the role of each element in enhancing the practice of Pilates.

In summary, the chapter "Preparation and Necessary Equipment" offers practical guidance on how to create an optimal training environment and select suitable equipment to maximize the benefits of Wall Pilates. Whether for beginners or experienced individuals, understanding how to prepare the space and use the tools correctly contributes to making the training more effective, safe, and rewarding.

Preparation

The "Preparation" segment within the chapter "Preparation and Necessary Equipment" focuses on organizing and setting up your training environment to maximize the benefits of your Wall Pilates exercises. Let's delve into the details of what this section entails:

Choosing the Ideal Location: Preparation begins with selecting the optimal location for your workout. This might involve choosing a quiet, well-lit space that is sufficiently large to perform exercises without obstacles. The ideal location contributes to creating an environment conducive to concentration and the effectiveness of exercises.

Space Organization: Proper space organization is essential. This involves arranging the area in a way that is free from distractions and safe for exercise. You may want to dedicate a specific space for your workout, ensuring it is clean and tidy.

Creating a Safe and Comfortable Environment: Ensure that the environment is safe and comfortable. Check for any obvious obstacles or hazards that could interfere with your practice. Consider adding elements, such as a mat, to make the surface more comfortable during floor exercises.

Eliminating External Distractions: Minimize external distractions. Turn off unnecessary electronic devices, and if possible, communicate to other family members or roommates that you are about to start your workout to avoid interruptions.

Mental Preparedness: Preparation is not just about the physical environment but also your mental state. Mentally prepare yourself to fully engage in the workout, focusing on the goals you want to achieve.

Considerations Before Starting the Workout: Before starting the exercises, take the time to warm up your body, perhaps with light stretching or dynamic movements. This prepares the muscles and improves flexibility, reducing the risk of injuries.

In summary, the "Preparation" section focuses on how to create a conducive environment for your Wall Pilates workout, both from a physical and mental standpoint, ensuring that each session is effective, safe, and rewarding.

Necessary Equipment

The "Necessary Equipment" section in the chapter "Preparation and Necessary Equipment" provides detailed guidance on the selection and correct use of tools and equipment required for practicing Wall Pilates. Let's explore in more detail what this section includes:

Mat: The mat is a fundamental element for performing floor exercises, providing comfortable support during workouts. Make sure to choose a mat that is thick enough to offer cushioning but also has enough grip to prevent slips.

Straps or Belts: Straps or belts are used to perform exercises involving arm and leg work. These tools can be adjustable to accommodate different needs and levels of flexibility.

Resistance Bands: Resistance bands are versatile tools that add resistance to movements, providing effective muscle work. They are often used for resistance exercises and to intensify training.

Optional Accessories: Depending on personal preferences and training goals, additional accessories such as Pilates balls, small weights, or elastic bands may be included. These accessories offer variety and can be used to increase the challenge of exercise.

Body Supports: In some exercises, it may be necessary to use body supports, such as pads or rolls, to provide comfort or facilitate certain movements.

Adaptability to Spaces: Consider how to adapt the equipment to your workout space. Some tools may require more space or a specific surface for optimal use.

In summary, the "Necessary Equipment" section provides essential information on the selection and correct use of tools to make the most of your Wall Pilates workout, ensuring both safety and effectiveness

CHAPTER 3: EFFECTIVE WARM-UP BEFORE THE WORKOUT

Introduction to the Chapter: Effective Warm-up Before the Workout

Welcome to the chapter dedicated to "Effective Warm-up Before the Workout." A proper warm-up is essential to optimally prepare the body for physical activity, maximizing the benefits of the training while reducing the risk of injuries. In this section, we will explore the importance of a well-structured warm-up before diving into your Wall Pilates exercises.

Warm-up is not just a routine phase but a crucial element in preparing muscles, joints, and the cardiorespiratory system for the impending activity. Together, we will navigate through a series of targeted exercises aimed at improving flexibility, increasing blood circulation, and activating key muscles involved in Wall Pilates.

Throughout this exploration, you will learn how to customize your warm-up based on your training goals and the expected intensity level. An effective warm-up not only enhances physical performance but also contributes to creating a deeper connection between the mind and body, preparing you for a Wall Pilates session that goes beyond mere physical practice.

Be ready to discover the art of effective warm-up, a valuable key to optimizing your Pilates experience and supporting your long-term physical well-being. Keep reading to embrace the full potential of your Wall Pilates workout.

Effective Warm-up Before the Workout

The chapter "Effective Warm-up Before the Workout" focuses on the importance of adequately preparing the body before engaging in more intense Wall Pilates exercises. Let's delve into the details of what this content entails:

Importance of Warm-up*:* The chapter begins by explaining why proper warm-up is crucial. It illustrates how warming up prepares the muscles, joints, and cardiorespiratory system for the impending activity. This crucial step not only optimizes the benefits of the workout but also helps reduce the risk of injuries.

Objectives of Warm-up: *I*t explains the specific objectives of the warm-up, which include improving flexibility, increasing blood circulation, and activating key muscles involved in Wall Pilates exercises. These goals aim to comprehensively prepare the body for movement.

Targeted Exercises: The section offers a series of targeted exercises that can be included in the warm-up. These exercises are designed to engage specific muscle groups, increase body temperature, and promote body awareness.

Customization of Warm-up: It encourages the customization of the warm-up based on individual training goals and the expected intensity level. This approach allows practitioners to adapt the warm-up to their own needs and physical conditions.

Benefits Beyond the Physical Aspect: It emphasizes that an effective warm-up goes beyond the physical aspect, contributing to establishing a deeper connection between the mind and body. This mental aspect mentally prepares the practitioner for a more comprehensive Pilates experience.

Role in Injury Prevention: It discusses the key role of warm-up in injury prevention, reducing the risk of muscle, tendon, or joint injuries during training.

In summary, the chapter "Effective Warm-up Before the Workout" provides a detailed guide on the importance of warm-up and how to structure it effectively to optimize the Wall Pilates experience.

Importance of Warm-Up

The importance of warming up is a fundamental concept in the context of any physical activity, including Wall Pilates. This section of the chapter emphasizes several key aspects related to the significance of warming up before engaging in more intense exercises. Let's delve into what this entails:

Muscular Preparation: Warming up prepares the muscles for the upcoming physical activity by gradually increasing their temperature. Warmed-up muscles respond better to exertion and are more flexible, reducing the risk of strains or injuries.

Increased Blood Circulation: During warming up, blood flow to the muscles increases, providing more oxygen and essential nutrients. This process promotes muscular readiness and enhances the body's ability to handle exertion.

Improved Flexibility: Warm-up exercises often include movements involving a wide range of joint and muscle motions. This contributes to increasing joint and muscle flexibility, making subsequent exercises more manageable.

Activation of the Cardiorespiratory System: Warming up isn't just about muscles; it also involves the cardiorespiratory system. Accelerated heart rate and improved breathing prepare the body for increased physical activity.

Enhanced Mind-Body Connection: Warming up provides an opportunity to mentally focus on the upcoming workout. This helps establish a better mind-body connection, improving awareness during exercises.

Reduced Risk of Injuries: Adequate warming up is crucial in injury prevention. Prepared muscles, tendons, and ligaments are less prone to damage during more intense efforts.

Improved Physical Performance: Overall, effective warming up enhances physical performance. Practitioners often experience increased strength, endurance, and coordination during subsequent exercises.

Understanding the importance of warming up before the workout is essential to optimize the benefits of physical activity, improve performance, and reduce the risk of injuries in the context of Wall Pilates.

Objectives of Warm-up

The "Objectives of Warm-up" section in the chapter "Effective Warm-up Before the Workout" focuses on the specific outcomes aimed to be achieved during the warm-up phase. Let's delve into the details of what these objectives entail:

Improving Flexibility: One of the primary goals of warm-up is to prepare muscles and joints by increasing their flexibility. Warm-up exercises aim to make muscle tissues more elastic, facilitating a broader range of motion during subsequent exercises.

Increasing Blood Circulation: An effective warm-up enhances blood flow to the muscles, providing them with a greater supply of oxygen and essential nutrients. This contributes to improving the efficiency of muscle work during the workout.

Activating Key Muscles: During warm-up, the focus is on activating specific muscles involved in subsequent exercises. This process prepares these muscles for the upcoming workload and enhances the mind-body connection.

Raising Body Temperature: A significant objective is to raise the body temperature. A warmer body becomes more flexible and responsive, reducing the risk of muscle strains or injuries during the workout.

Promoting Body Awareness: Warm-up is not only about the physical body but also the mind. Exercises aim to promote body awareness, enhancing the connection between the mind and body for more effective practice.

These objectives work synergistically to create an optimal bodily environment for training, improving performance, and reducing the risk of injuries. Overall, warm-up is an essential step to ensure that the body is ready to derive the maximum benefit from subsequent Wall Pilates exercises.

Targeted Exercises

The "Targeted Exercises" section of the chapter "Effective Warm-up Before the Workout" focuses on specific exercises performed during the warm-up phase. Let's delve into the details of what this part of the content entails:

Engagement of Specific Muscle Groups: Targeted exercises during warm-up are designed to engage specific muscle groups that will be involved in the main Wall Pilates workout. This ensures that these muscles are activated and ready for the upcoming activity.

Stretching and Activation Movements: Exercises may include stretching movements aimed at improving flexibility and range of motion. Simultaneously, they may actively involve muscles through contraction and relaxation movements, preparing them for a more intense workload.

Promotion of Stability and Balance: Some targeted exercises may focus on promoting stability and balance. These help prepare the body for Wall Pilates exercises that require control and coordination.

Dynamic and Controlled Movements: Warm-up exercises are often dynamic, involving controlled movements that contribute to increasing body temperature and improving movement fluidity.

Adaptability to Intensity Level: Targeted exercises can be adapted to the expected intensity level of the main workout. If the training program involves higher intensity, warm-up exercises can be designed accordingly.

Promotion of Mind-Body Connection: Targeted exercises are not only about physical preparation but also contribute to promoting the mind-body connection. This mental aspect is crucial for a more mindful and effective Pilates practice.

The "Targeted Exercises" section of the warm-up focuses on specific movements designed to prepare the body specifically for the upcoming Wall Pilates exercises, ensuring adequate muscle activation and a mindful connection between the mind and body.

Customization of Warm-up

The "Customization of the Warm-up" section in the chapter "Effective Warm-up Before the Workout" discusses the ability to tailor the warm-up phase based on individual needs and the desired intensity level. Let's explore in more detail what this content entails:

Adaptation to Training Goals: Customizing the warm-up allows practitioners to adjust the sequence of exercises based on specific training goals. If the aim is to focus on particular muscle groups or improve flexibility, one can select warm-up exercises accordingly.

Consideration of Fitness Level: Individuals with different fitness levels may require different warm-up approaches. Beginners might benefit from a more gradual and less intense warm-up phase compared to those with an advanced fitness level. Customization aligns with the level of physical preparedness.

Adoption of Exercise Variations: Customization may involve adopting variations of warm-up exercises. This allows modifying exercises based on personal preferences or any physical limitations, ensuring an effective and comfortable warm-up.

Variation in Duration: The duration of the warm-up can vary based on individual needs. In some cases, a longer warm-up may be necessary to fully prepare the body, while in other cases, a shorter warm-up may be sufficient.

Consideration of Daily Physical Conditions: Customization takes into account the individual's physical conditions on that particular day. If a practitioner feels particularly stiff or requires a more prolonged warm-up due to specific circumstances, they can adapt the sequence of exercises accordingly.

Flexibility in Approach: The customization of the warm-up reflects a certain flexibility in the approach. There is no one-size-fits-all warm-up sequence, and the ability to customize allows practitioners to tailor the warm-up phase to their specific needs.

In summary, "Customization of the Warm-up" provides the necessary flexibility to optimally tailor the warm-up phase to individual needs, ensuring that each practitioner is adequately prepared for the upcoming Wall Pilates training.

Benefits Beyond the Physical Aspect

The "Benefits Beyond the Physical Aspect" section in the chapter "Effective Warm-up Before the Workout" addresses the positive impacts that extend beyond the physical aspect during the warm-up phase. Let's explore in more detail what this content entails:

Promotion of Mind-Body Connection: An effective warm-up goes beyond merely preparing the body physically. It also involves promoting a deeper connection between the mind and body. Targeted exercises foster body awareness, helping create a stronger bond between physical activity and the mind.

Mental Preparation: The warm-up phase provides an opportunity to mentally prepare for the upcoming training. Through exercises involving concentration and mindfulness, practitioners can set aside external distractions and focus on the present moment.

Positive Emotional State: A well-structured warm-up can contribute to creating a positive emotional state. Increased body temperature and muscle activation can positively influence mood, fostering a conducive environment for training.

Stress Reduction: Through warm-up exercises that promote relaxation and awareness, the preparation phase can contribute to reducing mental stress. A more relaxed mind is often better prepared to face the physical challenges that follow in the Wall Pilates training.

Providing a Mental Break: The warm-up phase can serve as a mental break between everyday life and training. This interval allows practitioners to leave behind external concerns, creating mental space to focus on the upcoming activity.

The "Benefits Beyond the Physical Aspect" section highlights that warm-up is not only physical preparation but also an opportunity to prepare the mind, create a positive emotional state, and reduce stress, contributing to maximizing the Wall Pilates experience.

Role in Injury Prevention

The "Role in Injury Prevention" section in the chapter "Effective Warm-up Before the Workout" focuses on the importance of warm-up in preventing injuries during physical activity. Let's delve into the details of what this content entails:

Gradual Muscle Activation: During warm-up, muscles are gradually activated through targeted exercises. This process prepares the muscles for the more intense activity of the workout, reducing the risk of muscle injuries due to sudden strain on unprepared tissues.

Increase in Body Temperature: Warm-up contributes to an increase in body temperature, making muscles more flexible and elastic. This makes it less likely for strains or tears to occur during the execution of more demanding exercises.

Improved Blood Circulation: An increase in blood flow to the muscles during warm-up provides a greater supply of oxygen and nutrients. This improved circulation helps maintain muscle tissues healthy and reduces the likelihood of injuries related to inadequate blood supply.

Enhanced Joint Lubrication: Warm-up promotes the production of synovial fluid in the joints, improving their lubrication. Well-lubricated joints are less susceptible to trauma and injuries during wide and complex movements.

Increased Body Awareness: Warm-up exercises also promote increased body awareness, helping practitioners recognize any sensations of tension or discomfort. This awareness allows individuals to adapt their training based on their physical conditions, reducing the risk of injuries.

In summary, the "Role in Injury Prevention" section highlights how proper warm-up is crucial to safely prepare the body and reduce the risks of injuries during Wall Pilates training.

CHAPTER 4: WALL PILATES WORKOUTS FOR BEGINNERS

Introduction to the Chapter: Wall Pilates Workouts for Beginners

Welcome to the chapter dedicated to "Wall Pilates Workouts for Beginners." Whether you're new to the world of Pilates or already have some experience but are seeking a more accessible approach, you've made the right choice. This chapter is designed to guide you through a series of wall Pilates exercises specifically tailored for beginners.

Wall Pilates provides an excellent introduction to this workout method, combining the structural support of the wall with the fundamental principles of Pilates. Throughout this chapter, we'll explore gentle yet effective movements focused on building strength, flexibility, and body awareness.

You'll become familiar with key Pilates elements, learn basic positions, and discover how to use the wall as an ally in perfecting your technique. Each exercise is designed to accommodate your starting level, ensuring an approachable experience without excessive difficulty.

Get ready to experience the benefits of Wall Pilates, improving your posture, strengthening your body, and developing a profound awareness of your physical form. Put on comfortable clothing, make sure you have enough space, and get ready to dive into a Pilates practice that will accompany you on your physical and mental growth journey. Are you ready to embark on this journey towards a stronger, more flexible, and more aware version of yourself through Wall Pilates workouts for beginners?

The chapter "Wall Pilates Workouts for Beginners" is designed for those who are new to Pilates or seeking a more accessible approach to this form of exercise. Let's delve into the details of what this content entails:

Chapter Objectives: Specific objectives of the chapter are outlined, highlighting what beginners can expect to gain from these workouts. These objectives may include improvements in strength, flexibility, and body awareness.

Focus on Fundamental Principles: The fundamental principles of Pilates that will be applied during the workouts are introduced and explained. These principles include control, center (core), flow of movement, precision, breathing, and concentration.

Basic Positions: Basic positions used in various exercises are introduced. This may include starting positions, specific alignments, and establishing a solid foundation for the correct execution of exercises.

Gradual Approach: Emphasis is placed on a gradual approach to the exercises, encouraging beginners to progress at a comfortable pace and focus on the correct execution of exercises before increasing intensity.

Examples of Pilates Workouts for Beginners: This section will present some examples of Pilates Workouts for Beginners

In summary, "Wall Pilates Workouts for Beginners" offers a structured and accessible introduction to Wall Pilates, with a gradual approach, clear explanations of fundamental principles, and detailed exercise guidance to help beginners familiarize themselves with this form of training effectively and safely.

Chapter Objectives

The "Chapter Objectives" section introduces the specific purposes of the chapter dedicated to "Wall Pilates Workouts for Beginners." These objectives highlight what beginners can expect to gain from this part of the book. Specifically, the focus is on developments related to physical strength, flexibility, and body awareness. The aim is to guide readers through a structured journey that allows them to become acquainted with Wall Pilates pleasantly and progressively. Moreover, the goal is to create a safe and effective learning experience, with a particular emphasis on a clear understanding of the fundamental principles of Pilates and the establishment of a solid foundation for the correct execution of exercises.

Focus on Fundamental Principles

The "Focus on Fundamental Principles" section of the chapter on "Wall Pilates Workouts for Beginners" concentrates on introducing and explaining the fundamental principles of Pilates that will be applied during the proposed exercises. These principles are essential for an effective and mindful Pilates practice. Let's delve into the details of what this content entails:

The fundamental principles of Pilates include:

Control: The central idea is to perform exercises with precise control of movements. This involves constant awareness of how the body moves and responds to exercises, ensuring smooth and controlled executions.

Center (Core): Special emphasis is placed on strengthening the "center," referring to the abdominal region, pelvis, and lower back. This area is considered the focal point of movement in Pilates and contributes to stability and support during exercises.

Flow of Movement: Pilates encourages a continuous and controlled flow of movement, avoiding abrupt or disjointed motions. This principle aims to create seamless transitions between exercises, ensuring a smooth and uninterrupted experience.

Precision: Precision is crucial in executing exercises. Practitioners are encouraged to focus on details, such as correct posture and body alignment, to maximize benefits and prevent potential injuries.

Breathing: Breathing is integrated into movements. Controlled and coordinated breathing helps maintain body stability, promotes relaxation, and contributes to the harmonious flow of movements.

Concentration: Mental awareness is fundamental. Concentration during exercise execution allows for the connection of mind and body, enhancing the quality of performance and maximizing benefits.

These principles serve as a guide during Wall Pilates workouts for beginners, establishing a solid foundation for future, more advanced practice. By focusing on these fundamentals, participants can develop a profound awareness of their bodies and improve the quality of their movements over time.

Basic Positions

The "Basic Positions" section of the chapter on "Wall Pilates Workouts for Beginners" introduces and illustrates the fundamental positions that will be used during the exercises. These positions form the basis on which to build an effective Pilates practice. Let's explore what this content entails, including some examples of basic positions.

Neutral Spine Position: In this position, the spine is in a neutral alignment, maintaining its natural curvature. The feet are positioned shoulder-width apart, the knees are slightly bent, and the weight is evenly distributed.

Bridge Position: While lying on the back, with feet hip-width apart and knees bent, slowly lift the hips upward, creating a straight line from the shoulders to the feet.

Cat-Cow Position: In a tabletop position, with hands under the shoulders and knees under the hips, alternate between arching the back upward (cat position) and lowering the abdomen toward the floor (cow position).

Plank Position: From a tabletop position, extend the legs backward, maintaining a straight line from the head to the feet, supporting yourself on the palms of the hands and the tips of the toes.

Swan Position: Sitting with legs extended in front, place hands on the floor behind you and lift the torso upward, creating an arched curve.

Seated Lotus Position: Seated on the floor, cross the legs with feet resting on the opposite thighs, maintaining an upright posture.

These basic positions provide a solid foundation for performing Wall Pilates exercises correctly and effectively, helping develop strength, flexibility, and body awareness.

Gradual Approach

The "Gradual Approach" section in the chapter on "Wall Pilates Workouts for Beginners" emphasizes the importance of adopting a gradual approach during exercise practice. Let's explore in more detail what this content entails.

A gradual approach during Pilates workouts for beginners means:

Step-by-Step Progression: Instead of tackling advanced exercises from the beginning, it is recommended to start with simpler and more accessible movements. As familiarity with positions and fundamental principles grows, more complex exercises can be gradually introduced.

Adaptation at One's Own Pace: Every individual has a unique fitness level and familiarity with physical exercise. The gradual approach allows each practitioner to adapt workouts at their own pace, avoiding excessive fatigue or potential injuries.

Focus on Correct Execution: Rather than focusing on the quantity of exercise performed, emphasis is placed on correct execution. Gradual progression allows time to acquire proper technique, building a solid foundation for more advanced workouts in the future.

Body Awareness: The gradual approach encourages increased awareness of one's body during exercises. Practitioners learn to listen to the body's sensations, recognize individual limits, and adapt workouts accordingly.

Risk Reduction: Gradual increase in intensity reduces the risk of muscle or joint overloading. This contributes to keeping the practice safe and effective in the long run.

Appreciation of Progress: A gradual approach allows for appreciation and recognition of progress over time. As strength and flexibility are gained, this can further motivate the practitioner.

In summary, the gradual approach to Wall Pilates workouts for beginners aims to provide a solid and safe foundation for practice, promoting steady and sustainable progress over time.

Examples of Pilates Workouts for Beginners

Here are some examples of wall Pilates workouts suitable for beginners. These exercises are designed to develop strength, flexibility, and body awareness. Before starting any new workout program, make sure to get approval from your doctor, especially if you have pre-existing health conditions.

Exercise 1: "The Wall Roll Down"

Starting Position: Stand with your back against the wall, feet slightly wider than shoulder-width apart. Keep your head, spine, and heels against the wall.

Movement: Begin to slowly roll down towards the floor, sliding your back along the wall. Keep your abdominal muscles engaged and descend gradually towards the floor.

Objective: The goal is to reach a controlled squat position. Then, slowly rise back to the starting position.

Exercise 2: "Wall Squats"

Starting Position: Stand with your back against the wall and feet about shoulder-width apart.

Movement: Slowly descend into a squat position, keeping your back and head against the wall. Ensure that knees are aligned with ankles.

Objective: Maintain the squat position for a few seconds, then rise back to the starting position.

Exercise 3: "Leg Lifts"

Starting Position: Lie on your back with your legs against the wall, forming a right angle with the floor.

Movement: Lift your legs slowly upward along the wall, keeping your abdominal muscles engaged. Lower the legs slowly towards the floor without touching it.

Objective: The goal is to work on the strength of the abdominals and legs.

Exercise 4: "Wall Push-Ups"

Starting Position: Place your hands against the wall slightly wider than shoulder-width apart.

Movement: Perform a series of push-ups against the wall, keeping the body in a straight line. Keep the abdominal muscles engaged during the movement.

Objective: The goal is to work on the strength of the chest, shoulders, and arms.

Remember to perform each exercise slowly and with control, focusing on proper technique. Start with a few repetitions and gradually increase as you gain strength and endurance.

CHAPTER 5: MUSCLE STRENGTH ENHANCEMENT ADVANCED EXERCISES

The section "Muscular Strength Improvement: Advanced Exercises" within the context of "Wall Pilates Workouts for Beginners" addresses the progression to more challenging exercises aimed at enhancing muscular strength. Let's delve into the details of what this content entails:

Evolution of Exercises: After gaining confidence with basic exercises, this section introduces more advanced movements. The progression is designed to ensure participants can gradually build strength, flexibility, and muscular control.

Targeting Specific Muscle Groups: Advanced exercises often place greater emphasis on specific muscle groups, contributing to a more targeted development of strength. This may include specific exercises for glutes, abdominals, back, and other muscle groups.

Complexity of Movement: Advanced exercises may involve more complex and coordinated movements, requiring increased body awareness and finer muscular control. This stimulates the mind and body more comprehensively.

Advanced Wall Support Utilization: As participants engage in more advanced exercises, the wall can be utilized in more intricate ways to provide additional support and resistance. For instance, it may be leveraged for resistance exercises or as an unstable support surface, intensifying the training.

Increased Resistance: Advanced exercises may involve the use of specific equipment or modifiers to increase resistance and further challenge muscular strength. This could include the use of light weights, resistance bands, or Pilates balls.

Technique Oversight: With the complexity of exercises increasing, the section pays attention to proper technical execution. The guidance may include detailed tips on posture, alignment, and how to avoid common mistakes.

Gradual Transition: Despite the introduction of more advanced exercises, emphasis is placed on a gradual transition. This allows participants to progress at a pace that suits their capabilities, minimizing the risk of injuries.

In summary, the "Muscular Strength Improvement: Advanced Exercises" section provides a gradual roadmap for participants looking to push beyond basic exercises, focusing on progressively and safely enhancing muscular strength in the context of Wall Pilates.

Now here are some examples of advanced Pilates wall exercises. These exercises are designed to challenge strength, flexibility, and muscular control in a more advanced way. Before attempting advanced exercises, it is advisable to have a solid foundation with lower-level exercises and ensure that you are physically ready for the challenge.

Exercise 1: "Wall Plank with Leg Lifts"

Starting Position: Get into a plank position with hands placed against the wall and the body in a straight line.

Movement: Lift one leg slowly upward while maintaining the plank position. Alternate legs, focusing on core stability.

Objective: The goal is to work on core, arm, and leg strength.

Exercise 2: "Wall Bridge with Marching"

Starting Position: Lie on your back with your feet against the wall and knees bent.

Movement: Lift your hips slowly upward, forming a bridge.

Perform a "marching" movement by alternately lifting your knees toward your chest.

Objective: The objective is to engage the hamstrings, glutes, and core.

Exercise 3: "Wall Teaser"

Starting Position: Sit with your back against the wall, legs extended, and lifted off the ground.

Movement: Lean your torso backward slowly while keeping your legs lifted, forming a "V" with your body. Return slowly to the seated position.

Objective: The goal is to work on abdominal strength and body control.

Exercise 4: "Wall Saw"

Starting Position: Sit with legs apart, feet against the wall, and reach arms forward.

Movement: Rotate the torso and arms to one side, attempting to touch the opposite foot. Return to the center and repeat on the opposite side.

Objective: The objective is to engage the obliques and improve spinal flexibility.

Remember to perform these exercises carefully, focus on proper technique, and maintain control during each movement. Adjust the difficulty based on your fitness level, and if in doubt, consult a Pilates instructor for personalized guidance.

CHAPTER 6: FOCUS ON FLEXIBILITY AND JOINT MOBILITY

The chapter "Focus on Flexibility and Joint Mobility" is centered on the importance of developing and maintaining muscle flexibility and joint mobility within the context of wall Pilates workouts.

Muscle flexibility involves the ability to stretch muscles, improving the range of motion, while joint mobility refers to the ability to move joints through their full range of motion. These aspects not only contribute to improved posture and body alignment but are crucial for reducing the risk of muscle and joint injuries, promoting blood circulation, and increasing freedom of movement.

The chapter introduces specific wall Pilates exercises designed to enhance flexibility and joint mobility. These exercises include active stretching practices involving muscle contraction during relaxation and dynamic stretching encouraging controlled movement through a range of motions.

Special emphasis is placed on using the wall as support during flexibility exercises. This not only enhances stability but can also be leveraged to provide gradual resistance during muscle relaxation, intensifying the effectiveness of the training. Now here are some examples of this kind of exercise.

"Stretch and Reach" at the Wall: Stand with the side of your body facing the wall, raise one arm along the wall, and stretch your body in the opposite direction. This exercise involves lateral flexibility of the spine.

"Butterfly Stretch" with Wall Support: Sit with your back against the wall, bring the soles of your feet together, and let your knees drop towards the floor. The wall provides additional support as you work on hip and groin flexibility.

"Wall Assisted Forward Fold": Stand a few steps away from the wall, place your hands at shoulder height, and push your hips back, bending your body forward. The wall offers support during the forward bend to improve leg and lower back flexibility.

"Lunging Hip Flexor Stretch" at the Wall: Place one foot in front of the other with the back knee bent, and lean slightly forward. The wall can be used to maintain balance as you work on flexibility in the front of the thigh and hip.

"Wall Supported Leg Swings": Support one hand against the wall and swing one leg forward and backward. This dynamic exercise helps increase hip mobility and flexibility in the back of the leg.

"Seated Spinal Twist" with Wall Support: Sit with legs extended, rotate the torso to one side, and use the wall for support to deepen the spinal twist.

"Quad Stretch" at the Wall: Stand with the wall behind you, bend one leg bringing the heel towards the buttocks, and grab the ankle. This exercise aims to improve flexibility in the quadriceps.

"Supported Chest Opener" at the Wall: Stand close to the wall, extend one arm to the side, and rotate the torso, using the wall for support to open the chest.

These examples represent a variety of exercises that can be integrated into a wall Pilates routine, focusing on flexibility and joint mobility. The presence of the wall provides support and allows for greater control during the execution of exercises. It is recommended to perform each exercise slowly, focusing on proper technique, and adjusting the intensity based on individual needs and capabilities.

CHAPTER 7: BALANCE AND COORDINATION IN WALL PILATES

The chapter "Balance and Coordination in Wall Pilates" focuses on the importance of developing and refining balance and coordination through Pilates workouts using the support of the wall. Let's delve into the topics that will be addressed in this chapter:

Definition of Balance and Coordination

Balance: The ability to maintain control of the body and position during movement.

Coordination: The ability to execute fluid and controlled movements involving multiple parts of the body.

Benefits of Balance and Coordination in Wall Pilates

Reduction of the risk of falls and injuries by developing stability.

Improvement of body awareness and motor control.

Increase in strength in stabilizing muscles.

Integration of Specific Exercises

Introduction of wall Pilates exercises designed to enhance balance, often incorporating various positions and postures.

Use of the wall as a reference point to encourage control during exercises.

Dynamic Balance Exercises

Introduction of exercises involving dynamic movements, such as weight shifts and load transfers, to improve balance in moving situations.

Coordination and Movement Sequences

Inclusion of complex movement sequences requiring precise coordination between body parts.

Gradual progression of sequences to acclimate users to more complex tasks.

Use of the Wall for Progressive Support

Utilization of the wall as gradual support for more advanced balance exercises.

Tips on using the wall to adjust the difficulty of exercises based on proficiency level.

Progression of Balance Exercises

Suggestions on how to progressively increase the complexity and duration of balance exercises.

Advice on modifying exercises based on individual needs.

Integration with Pilates Principles

Emphasis on how fundamental Pilates principles, such as control, precision, and fluidity of movement, contribute to balance and coordination.

Practical Application in Daily Life

Advice on how skills developed in wall Pilates can be applied in daily activities, improving stability and coordination.

Muscle Strengthening Sessions for Stability

Specific exercises targeting the strengthening of fundamental stabilizing muscles for supporting balance.

Visual and Sensory Feedback

Discussion on the importance of utilizing visual and sensory feedback to improve balance and coordination.

Problem-Solving for Balance Issues

Strategies and specific exercises to address any difficulties or individual imbalances.

This chapter aims to provide a thorough understanding of how balance and coordination can be developed and strengthened through Wall Pilates. Through a series of specific exercises, gradual progressions, and practical advice, users can enhance their stability, motor control, and coordination, bringing tangible benefits to their daily lives.

Definition of Balance and Coordination

The concept of "Balance" in the context of Wall Pilates refers to the ability to maintain control of the body and position during movement. Balance is a fundamental component of physical development, contributing to stability and posture. In Pilates, this means being able to perform exercises in different positions while maintaining precise control without losing balance.

On the other hand, "Coordination" involves the ability to execute fluid and controlled movements involving multiple parts of the body simultaneously. In Wall Pilates, coordination is crucial because many exercises require the harmonious integration of movements of the upper and lower limbs, as well as the synchronization of various muscle actions.

Developing good balance and coordination offers several benefits. Firstly, it reduces the risk of falls and injuries, as increased stability allows for safer movements. Additionally, it enhances body awareness, enabling individuals to better perceive their bodies in space and respond appropriately to changes in posture.

During Wall Pilates workouts, exercises are designed to improve these abilities. This may include movements involving the shifting of body weight from one side to another, exercises that require maintaining unstable positions, and sequences of movements that challenge coordination.

Furthermore, using the wall as a reference point contributes to strengthening balance by providing stable support. This is particularly useful for those developing these skills, allowing them to progress gradually through more complex exercises.

Overall, the definition of balance and coordination in the context of Wall Pilates emphasizes the importance of developing a solid foundation of body control and harmonious movements. The goal is to integrate these principles into daily practice, bringing tangible benefits to stability, coordination, and overall well-being.

Benefits of Balance and Coordination in Wall Pilates

The benefits of developing balance and coordination in the context of Wall Pilates are manifold and significantly contribute to physical well-being and the quality of movement. Without listing, let's explore in more detail how these aspects positively impact the training experience:

Stability and Safety: The development of balance through Wall Pilates contributes to increased body stability. This translates into a sense of safety during exercise execution, reducing the risk of falls or loss of control. A stable base provides a secure platform for exploring more complex movements.

Improved Motor Control: Wall Pilates aims to refine motor control, the ability to coordinate and regulate body movements precisely. This involves greater awareness of muscle actions and how the body responds to different stimuli. Improved motor control is reflected not only in exercises but also in daily activities.

Increased Strength in Stabilizing Muscles: Balance exercises in Wall Pilates actively engage in stabilizing muscles. These often-neglected muscles are essential for maintaining posture, supporting joints, and preventing injuries. Developing strength in these muscles contributes to a more solid and resilient body structure.

Enhancement of Proprioception: Practicing Wall Pilates promotes the refinement of proprioception, the ability to perceive the position and movement of the body in space without relying excessively on sight. This sensory development is essential for conscious and precise movement, allowing automatic adjustment of posture and balance.

Adaptability in Movements: Wall Pilates training encourages the body's adaptability to different situations and stimuli. Exercises challenge the body to react and adjust its balance in response to variations in positions and movement dynamics. This improves the body's ability to handle a broader range of daily and sports activities.

Body and Mental Awareness: The pursuit of balance requires intensified awareness of both the body and the mind. In Wall Pilates, individuals learn to focus on the present, listen to their bodies, and respond to challenges with attention. This leads to an overall increase in awareness, creating a deeper connection between mind and body.

Posture Improvement: The development of balance goes hand in hand with an improvement in posture. Targeted exercises in Wall Pilates help strengthen the muscles supporting the spine and promote an upright and aligned posture. Correct posture contributes to preventing muscle pains and tension.

In summary, the benefits of developing balance and coordination in Wall Pilates are inherently linked to an improvement in stability, motor control, strength in stabilizing muscles, and body and mental awareness. These elements result in a more comprehensive training experience and the ability to apply the acquired benefits to daily activities.

Integration of Specific Exercises

In the context of Wall Pilates, the "Integration of Specific Exercises" refers to the targeted incorporation of workout routines that focus on and enhance balance using the wall as a support. These exercises are designed to challenge the body in ways that require heightened awareness of one's balance while concurrently developing strength, flexibility, and coordination.

Examples of Pilates Exercises to Improve Balance

"Wall Plank":

Place hands on the wall at shoulder level and align the body in a plank position. This exercise engages the entire body, requiring stability in the core and shoulders.

"Single Leg Wall Squat":

Lean against the wall and lower the body into a squat with one leg lifted. This exercise develops leg strength and requires significant control to maintain balance.

"Wall Ball Roll Down":

Lean against the wall with a ball between your back and the wall. Slowly perform a roll down to the floor and then rise back up. This exercise improves flexibility and engages stabilizing muscles.

"One-Legged Wall Push-Up":

Perform a push-up with one leg raised against the wall. This exercise requires stability in the upper body and develops strength in the core muscles.

"Wall Sit with Leg Lifts":

Sit with your back against the wall and lift one leg at a time. This exercise engages leg muscles and requires balance to maintain the "wall sit" position.

"Wall Bridge":

Lie on your back with your feet against the wall and lift the hips. This exercise strengthens the lower back, and glutes, and requires stability in the core.

"Toe Taps on the Wall":

Lie down with your back on the floor and legs extended up against the wall. Lightly tap the floor with the tips of your toes and return to the starting position. This exercise engages the abdominal muscles and improves coordination.

"Wall Roll-Up":

Sit with your back against the wall, extend your legs, and slowly reach for your toes. This exercise works on spinal flexibility and requires precise core control.

"Side Plank with Leg Lift":

Support the body on one side with one arm against the wall, lifting one leg. This exercise targets the lateral muscles and improves lateral balance.

"Wall Mermaid Stretch":

Sit with one side against the wall, bending the knees and reaching the arm above the head toward the wall. This exercise increases lateral flexibility and engages the abdominal muscles.

The integration of these specific exercises into the Wall Pilates program provides a comprehensive approach to improving balance, engaging different muscle groups, and developing a deeper awareness of the body during exercise.

Dynamic Balance Exercises

In the context of Wall Pilates, "Dynamic Balance Exercises" focus on performing movements that engage balance in dynamic situations. These exercises aim to develop the body's ability to maintain stability during controlled and fluid movements, often challenging the body to adapt to changes in positions and directions.

Examples of Dynamic Balance Exercises:

"Dynamic Lunges with Wall Touch":

Perform dynamic lunges with one leg extended backward, touching the wall with the opposite hand. This exercise develops balance and leg strength.

"Wall Tap Plank":

From a plank position, alternately tap the wall with each hand. This exercise engages the core and requires lateral balance control.

"Dynamic Side Leg Lifts":

Stand sideways to the wall and dynamically lift the leg laterally. This exercise targets lateral muscles and improves balance.

"Wall Roll with Knee Tuck":

Place hands on the wall in a plank position. Roll the knees toward the chest and then extend them back. This exercise develops control and balance.

"Dynamic Wall Squat Jumps":

Perform dynamic squats against the wall with controlled jumps. This exercise engages leg muscles and requires balance during the jump.

"Wall Mountain Climbers":

From a plank position with hands against the wall, alternately bring knees toward the chest. This exercise improves core stability and balance.

"Dynamic Wall Push-Ups":

Perform dynamic push-ups against the wall with dynamic movements. This exercise engages the upper body and requires stability and control.

"Wall Balance Leg Swings":

Balance on one leg with wall support and swing the other leg laterally. This exercise improves balance and coordination.

"Dynamic Wall Plank with Leg Lifts":

From a plank position with hands against the wall, alternately lift the legs. This exercise strengthens the core and develops balance and coordination.

"Wall Side Plank Twists":

In a side plank position with wall support, perform twists by bringing the arm toward the ceiling. This exercise improves balance and engages oblique muscles.

Dynamic balance exercises in Wall Pilates offer an advanced mode to develop stability, strength, and coordination in more dynamic scenarios. These movements continuously challenge the body to adapt, providing a comprehensive and functional workout.

Coordination and Movement Sequences

In the context of Wall Pilates, "Coordination and Movement Sequences" refer to the practice of exercises that require precise coordination between different parts of the body during specific sequences of movements. This aspect aims to develop the body's ability to perform fluid and controlled movements, harmoniously coordinating muscle actions and enhancing body awareness.

Key Objectives

Precision in Movements: The goal is to execute each movement with precision, controlling the pace and body position. This requires particular attention to detail and the quality of execution.

Articulated Sequences: Movement sequences are designed to flow seamlessly from one exercise to another. This develops the body's ability to adapt without abrupt interruptions, enhancing fluidity in movements.

Full Body Engagement: Sequences are designed to engage different parts of the body simultaneously, requiring precise coordination between the upper and lower body, as well as engaging the core.

Enhancement of Body Awareness: Performing sequences requires increased awareness of body movements in space. This develops a deeper connection between mind and body, improving the quality of the workout.

Examples of Coordination and Movement Sequence Exercises:

"Wall Squat to Leg Lift to Side Kick":

Combine a wall squat with lifting one leg and executing a controlled sidekick. This exercise requires coordination between leg and core actions.

"Dynamic Wall Plank to Pike Stretch":

From a plank position, perform a fluid upward movement, raising the hips into a "V" position. This sequence engages the core and requires coordination in movements.

"Wall Roll-Up to Teaser":

Combine the wall roll-up with the teaser, lifting both legs and torso. This exercise demands precision in movements and coordination between the upper and lower body.

"Leg Circles with Arm Movements":

Execute leg circles while coordinating movements with the arms. This exercise engages various body parts simultaneously.

"Wall Plank to Side Plank Transitions":

Alternate between wall plank and side plank, requiring a smooth transition and coordination between positions. The integration of exercises focused on coordination and movement sequences in Wall Pilates offers an advanced training mode that develops precision in movements and the body's ability to execute harmonious sequences with increased awareness and control.

Use of the Wall for Progressive Support

In the context of Wall Pilates, the "Progressive Use of the Wall for Support" refers to the practice of integrating the wall as a gradual support during exercise execution. This approach allows practitioners to progressively develop strength, stability, and flexibility by utilizing the wall as an adjustable support aid.
Gradual Approach:

Support for Beginners: Begin by offering the wall as support for basic exercises. For example, during lunges or squats, the wall can provide extra stability for those developing leg strength.

Progression in Balance: As strength and stability improve, the wall can be used more subtly for exercises involving balance. For instance, wall support can be lightened during single-leg positions.

Support for Advanced Exercises: For more advanced exercises requiring increased core strength or specific positioning, the wall can serve as a reference point to maintain proper form and facilitate a safe progression.

Benefits of Using the Wall

Improvement of Form: The wall serves as a visual and physical guide to maintaining correct form during exercises, helping prevent poor postural habits.

Increased Flexibility: For stretching exercises or movements involving flexibility, the wall can be used to gradually increase the range of motion in a controlled manner.

Psychological Support: By providing gradual support, the wall can contribute to improving the confidence of practitioners, allowing them to challenge themselves safely and progress in their fitness journeys.

Adaptability to Various Abilities: The use of the wall allows instructors to tailor exercises to different abilities and fitness levels, making Pilates accessible to a wide range of participants.

Progression of Balance Exercises

The "Progression of Balance Exercises" in the context of Wall Pilates refers to the gradual approach to increasing the complexity and intensity of exercises aimed at improving body balance. This process allows practitioners to gradually develop the strength and stability needed to tackle increasingly advanced challenges in maintaining position and control during balance exercises.

Phases of Progression

Stable Base: Begin with exercises that offer a stable base. For example, perform balance exercises with both feet in contact with the ground or use the wall for light support.

Gradual Support Reduction: Progressively reduce the support provided by the wall or other aids during balance exercises. This challenges the body to adapt and use stabilizing muscles more intensely.

Variety in Contact Points: Introduce variations in contact points with the ground. For example, perform balance exercises with only one foot on the ground or with different combinations of contacts such as toes, heels, or the edge of the foot.

Dynamic Movements: Progress towards balance exercises involving dynamic movements. For instance, perform lunges or lateral bends while maintaining balance in more challenging positions.

Eyes Closed: Advance gradually by introducing balance exercises with closed eyes. This adds challenge, requiring increased reliance on the sense of body position.

Benefits of Progression of Balance Exercises

Development of Stabilizing Strength: Progression allows stabilizing muscles to adapt and develop gradually, contributing to overall body strength improvement.

Increased Body Awareness: Progressive balance exercises increase body awareness, enhancing the connection between mind and body.

Reduced Risk of Injuries: Improving balance reduces the risk of injuries related to loss of stability, especially in daily or sports-related situations.

Posture Improvement: Progressive balance contributes to posture improvement by developing awareness of body position in space.

Examples of Progressive Balance Exercises:

"Wall-Supported Leg Lift":

Lift one leg with wall support, focusing on the stability of the supporting leg.

"Single-Leg Balance":

Maintain balance on one leg without support to increase stability challenges.

"Dynamic Lunges":

Perform dynamic lunges, adding a movement element to the traditional balance exercise.

"Toe Taps":

From a balance position, gently tap the ground with the toe, varying the contact points.

"Eyes-Closed Balance":

Try balance exercises with closed eyes to further challenge the sense of body position.

The progression of balance exercises in Wall Pilates provides a structured path to enhance balance, allowing a gradual transition to more advanced challenges and promoting better body awareness.

Integration with Pilates Principles

"Integration with Pilates Principles" in the context of Wall Pilates refers to the harmonious fusion of traditional Pilates exercises with the use of the wall as an additional aid. This approach aims to combine the unique benefits of wall training with the fundamental principles of Pilates, creating a synergistic practice that emphasizes control, precision, and body awareness. Now we repeat for the contest of this chapter, the foundations of pilates principles:

Control: Maintain precise control during each movement, using the wall to support and enhance your execution.

Precision: Focus on the precision of movements, integrating the wall as a reference to ensure proper form and alignment.

Center (Core): Engage the center of the body, the core, specifically during exercises, using the wall as support to strengthen your core.

Flow of Movement: Create a smooth flow between exercises, using the wall to facilitate transitions and maintain a continuous connection between different positions.

Precision: Focus on the precision of movements, integrating the wall as a reference to ensure proper form and alignment.

Integrating the Wall into Pilates Principles:

Spinal Support: The wall can be used as support to maintain proper spinal alignment during exercises such as the roll-up or spinal extension.

Core Strength Development: Integrate the wall into specific core exercises, providing gradual support for core muscle strengthening.

Increased Body Awareness: Use the wall as a guide to improve body awareness, focusing on the sensation and precise control of movements.

Position Variations: Leverage the wall to vary body position during exercises, adding challenges and requiring adaptations in line with Pilates principles.

Gradual Resistance Addition: Integrate the wall to add gradual resistance to exercises, promoting the development of strength in harmony with Pilates principles.

The integration with Pilates principles in Wall Pilates offers a comprehensive approach that combines the solidity of traditional exercises with the innovation of wall training, creating a practice that resonates with the fundamental aspects of Pilates.

Practical Application in Daily Life

"Practical Application in Daily Life" in the context of Wall Pilates refers to the transferability of exercises and principles learned during wall training sessions into everyday life. This aspect aims to demonstrate how the teachings of Wall Pilates can be integrated into daily routines to improve posture, strength, flexibility, and overall well-being.

Connection with Daily Activities: Optimal Posture: Apply the learned principles of spinal alignment from Wall Pilates to maintain optimal posture while engaging in daily activities such as sitting at the computer or lifting heavy objects.

Controlled Movements: Use the awareness of controlled movements acquired during Wall Pilates exercises to perform more controlled and safe movements during daily activities.

Core Integration: Engage the core in daily activities, applying the strength and stability developed through Wall Pilates exercises. This can include activities like house cleaning or lifting grocery bags.

Mindful Breathing: Maintain mindful breathing during daily activities, using the deep and controlled breathing learned in Wall Pilates to reduce stress and improve respiratory efficiency.

Agility and Flexibility: Apply agility and flexibility exercises from Wall Pilates when performing daily movements such as bending to pick something up or reaching for objects in hard-to-reach places.

Benefits of Practical Application:

Injury Prevention: Applying Wall Pilates principles in daily activities contributes to injury prevention by improving body awareness and stabilizing strength.

Overall Well-being Improvement: Integrating Wall Pilates teachings into daily life promotes overall well-being by improving posture, reducing muscle tension, and enhancing mobility.

Efficiency in Movements: Practical application helps make movements more efficient and ergonomic, reducing unnecessary effort and improving fluidity in movements.

Body Awareness: Using Wall Pilates principles in daily activities develops increased body awareness, promoting better balance and coordination.

Continuity in Progress: Consistent application helps maintain and solidify the progress achieved during Wall Pilates sessions in the long term.

The goal of practical application in daily life is to transform the teachings of Wall Pilates from an isolated training experience into an integrated element in everyday life, bringing tangible and lasting benefits.

Muscle Strengthening Sessions for Stability

The "Muscle Strengthening Sessions for Stability" in the context of Wall Pilates refers to a series of targeted exercises designed to strengthen specific muscle groups, thus enhancing overall body stability. These sessions focus on using the wall as support to provide resistance and additional stimulus during exercises, contributing to the development of a strong and stable muscular foundation.

Fundamental Principles of the Sessions:

Core Engagement: Each exercise aims to actively engage core muscles, strengthening the abdominals, obliques, and lower back muscles to improve trunk stability.

Wall Utilization for Resistance: The wall is used as support and a point of resistance for exercises involving both the upper and lower body, intensifying muscular efforts.

Gradual Progression: Gradual progression of exercises allows participants to adapt progressively to new challenges, ensuring a balanced development of strength and stability.

Movement Control: Each movement is executed with careful control, emphasizing the quality of movement over quantity to maximize muscular benefits.

Focus on Specific Muscle Groups: The sessions concentrate on specific muscle groups, including often-neglected ones, to ensure a well-rounded development of muscle strength and stability.

Examples of Exercises:

"Wall Squats": Perform squats with wall support to strengthen the lower body, including quadriceps, glutes, and abdominal muscles.

"Wall Push-Ups": Execute push-ups with hands against the wall to strengthen the upper body, focusing on the shoulders, chest, and triceps.

"Leg Raises with Wall Support": Lift legs with wall support to strengthen lower abdominals and improve core stability.

"Wall Plank": Perform a plank with elbows resting against the wall to actively engage abdominal and stabilizing muscles.

"Wall Bridge": Execute a bridge with feet against the wall to work on the posterior thigh muscles and glutes.

Benefits of Muscle Strengthening Sessions for Stability:

Increased Overall Strength: Contribute to developing improved overall strength, engaging both the upper and lower body.

Enhanced Core Stability: Significantly strengthen core muscles, improving trunk stability and posture.

Prevention of Overexertion: Strengthen stabilizing muscles, helping to prevent overexertion and injuries during daily activities.

Exercise Versatility: The versatility of exercises allows for a variety of options to adapt sessions based on fitness levels and individual needs.

Continuous Integration: Easily integrated into existing workout routines, providing a solid foundation for further strength and stability development.

Muscle strengthening sessions for stability in Wall Pilates offer a targeted approach to improving muscle strength and body stability, effectively incorporating wall support into various exercises.

Visual and Sensory Feedback

"Visual and Sensory Feedback" in the context of Wall Pilates refers to the awareness and perception stimulated through the use of the wall as a reference point during exercises. This approach aims to enhance precision, body awareness, and the effectiveness of exercise execution by incorporating both visual and sensory feedback.

Key Elements of Visual and Sensory Feedback:

Posture Observation: Use the wall as a visual reference to observe your posture during exercises, ensuring proper alignment of the spine and joints.

Movement Monitoring: Closely observe body movements about the wall, providing immediate feedback on the correct execution of exercises and body alignment.

Position Corrections: Use visual feedback to correct body positions, improving the precision and effectiveness of exercises by Pilates principles.

Tactile Sensations: Leverage tactile sensations generated by contact with the wall to enhance body awareness, focusing on how the body interacts with the support provided by the wall.

Breathing Focus: Use visual feedback to monitor the synchronization of breathing with movements, ensuring controlled and coordinated breathing.

Benefits of Visual and Sensory Feedback:

Alignment Improvement: Visual feedback helps maintain proper alignment, contributing to preventing incorrect postures and muscle tensions.

Increased Body Awareness: Attention to sensory feedback develops greater body awareness, allowing a deeper understanding of movements and bodily sensations.

Immediate Corrections: Visual feedback allows for immediate corrections during exercises, ensuring that the body moves appropriately and safely.

Mind-Body Connection: Mindful use of visual and sensory feedback promotes a stronger connection between the mind and body during exercise execution.

Enhanced Effectiveness: Integrating visual and sensory feedback makes exercises more effective, enabling more precise control movements and greater attention to alignment.

The incorporation of visual and sensory feedback in Wall Pilates emphasizes the importance of awareness during exercises, contributing to optimizing movement quality and maximizing the benefits of training.

Problem-Solving for Balance Issues

"Balance Problem Solving" in the context of Wall Pilates focuses on targeted strategies and exercises to enhance body stability and address any challenges related to balance. This aspect is particularly relevant as the use of the wall as support provides a unique opportunity to develop a stable foundation, refine body control, and address balance-related difficulties. Approach to Balance Problem Solving:

Balance Analysis: Assess your ability to maintain balance during exercises, identifying any areas of weakness or instability.

Focus on the Core: Concentrate on actively engaging the core to stabilize the trunk and improve coordination of movements about the wall.

Gradual Progression of Exercises: Introduce balance exercises gradually, starting with simpler positions and progressing gradually to progressively challenge your stability.

Use of the Wall as a Reference Point: Utilize the wall as a reference point to stabilize yourself during balance exercises, allowing for increased safety and confidence.

Exploration of Different Positions: Experiment with various body positions about the wall, encouraging a comprehensive understanding of your balance and areas that require attention.

Examples of Balance Problem-Solving Exercises:

"One-Legged Wall Stand": Lift one leg at a time while maintaining contact with the wall, developing leg strength and improving balance.

"Wall Plank with Leg Lifts": Perform a plank with alternately lifted legs, improving core stability and developing strength in the arms and legs.

"Wall Squats with Rotation": Execute squats with wall support, incorporating torso rotation to enhance stability and flexibility.

"Wall Lunges": Perform lunges while maintaining contact with the wall, developing leg strength and improving coordination.

"Single Leg Wall Bridge": Execute the bridge on one leg at a time, improving core stability and developing strength in the posterior thigh muscles and glutes.

Benefits of Balance Problem Solving:

Improved Stability: Addressing and solving balance challenges contributes to improving overall body stability.

Increased Strength and Coordination: Working on balanced problem-solving promotes the development of muscle strength and coordination.

Fall Prevention: Improving balance is crucial for fall prevention, especially in older adults.

Body Awareness: Attention to balance enhances greater body awareness, improving spatial perception and coordination.

Safety and Confidence: Addressing and solving balance challenges with the support of the wall builds safety and confidence in one's movements.

The approach to balance problem-solving in Wall Pilates aims to create a stable foundation, developing strength, coordination, and confidence in movements related to balance.

CHAPTER 8: WALL PILATES ROUTINES FOR MUSCLE TONING

The "Wall Pilates Routine for Muscle Toning" is a targeted approach that leverages the support of the wall to develop and tone specific muscle groups. This routine focuses on combining the fundamental principles of Pilates with the strategic use of the wall, providing an effective and targeted workout experience for muscle toning.

Approach to Muscle Toning:

Core Engagement: Each exercise is designed to activate the core, engaging the abdominals and obliques to stabilize the trunk.

Use of the Wall for Resistance: The wall is used as a point of resistance to intensify muscle efforts, contributing to toning arms, legs, and the abdominal area.

Variety of Movements: The routine includes a variety of movements involving different muscle groups, ensuring comprehensive muscle toning throughout the body.

Gradual Progression: Exercises are structured with a gradual progression, allowing anyone, from beginners to advanced participants, to join and progress.

Concentration and Precision: Emphasis is placed on concentration and precision in executing exercises, maximizing benefits, and reducing the risk of injuries.

Examples of Muscle Toning Exercises:

"Wall Squats with Bicep Curls": Perform squats with wall support, simultaneously incorporating bicep curls with light weights to tone legs and arms.

"Leg Lifts with Wall Support": Lift legs with the wall as support, toning lower abdominals and strengthening the core.

"Triceps Dips against the Wall": Execute triceps dips against the wall to work on arm muscles and upper body.

"Wall Plank with Leg Extensions": Perform a plank with leg extensions to actively engage the core and tone the lower limbs.

"Wall Push-Ups with Knee Tucks": Combine wall push-ups with knee tucks for a complete workout of chest, shoulders, and abs.

Benefits of Muscle Toning Routine:

Balanced Muscle Development: The routine aims to tone various muscle groups in a balanced manner, promoting harmonious development.

Improved Functional Strength: Exercises are designed to enhance functional strength, contributing to better performance in daily activities.

Muscle Definition: Through wall resistance, the routine aims to define and sculpt muscles, improving overall physical appearance.

Added Flexibility and Stability: Integrating Pilates principles, the routine not only tones but also contributes to improving flexibility and stability.

Adaptability to Different Levels: The gradual progression of exercises allows participants of different levels to adapt the routine to their abilities and goals.

The "Wall Pilates Routine for Muscle Toning" offers a versatile and effective approach for those looking to build strength and muscle definition, creatively incorporating wall support into various exercises.

CHAPTER 9: WEIGHT MANAGEMENT AND CARDIOVASCULAR WORKOUTS

Weight management through cardiovascular workouts is a fundamental aspect of a comprehensive fitness program. This approach combines targeted exercises to improve cardiovascular health with strategies aimed at controlling body weight. Here's a detailed overview of the topic:

Importance of Weight Management:

Cardiovascular Health: Maintaining a healthy body weight is crucial for the health of the heart and blood vessels, reducing the risk of cardiovascular diseases.

Energy Balance: Weight management revolves around the balance between energy consumed through diet and energy burned through physical activity.

Disease Control: Maintaining an appropriate body weight contributes to the prevention of conditions such as type 2 diabetes and hypertension.

Role of Cardiovascular Workouts:

Calorie Burning: Cardiovascular exercises like running, cycling, and swimming are effective in burning calories, and facilitating weight loss and weight maintenance.

Metabolism Boost: Cardiovascular training can increase metabolism, contributing to greater calorie burning even at rest.

Promotion of Cardiovascular Health: Cardiovascular exercises improve blood circulation, cardiac endurance, and lung capacity, promoting optimal cardiovascular health.

Cardiovascular Training Strategies for Weight Management:

Aerobic Exercises: Include activities like running, swimming, cycling, and aerobics to promote increased heart rate and calorie expenditure.

Interval Training: Alternate short bursts of high intensity with recovery periods to maximize calorie burning and improve endurance.

Long-Duration Aerobic Activities: Engage in long-duration aerobic activities, such as extended walks or jogging sessions, to support gradual weight loss.

Important Considerations:

Balanced Nutrition: Pair cardiovascular workouts with a balanced diet for optimal results in weight management.

Consistency and Gradual Progression: Maintain a regular cardiovascular workout routine and progress gradually to avoid injuries and consistently improve performance.

Medical Consultation: Before starting an intense workout program, it's advisable to consult with a medical professional to ensure it is safe and suitable for individual physical conditions.

Weight management through cardiovascular workouts is a comprehensive approach that not only contributes to weight loss but also promotes better cardiovascular and overall health.

Additionally, cardiovascular training and Pilates are two complementary fitness approaches, each with its distinct benefits. Their combination can form a balanced workout program that promotes overall health and well-being. Here's an explanation of the relationship between cardiovascular training and Pilates:

Integration for Balance: Cardiovascular training can be integrated with Pilates to achieve a balance between high-intensity activities and those concentrating on strength and control.

Warm-Up and Cool-Down: A short cardiovascular workout can serve as a warm-up before a Pilates session, while light cardiovascular training can be incorporated as a cool-down afterward.

Holistic Fitness Program: Combining both provides a comprehensive overview, with cardiovascular training addressing heart health and calorie expenditure, and Pilates focusing on strength, flexibility, and muscle control.

Adaptability to Individual Needs: The relationship between the two can vary based on individual needs and goals, creating a personalized and sustainable fitness program over time.

The key is to find a balance between these two training modalities, customizing the approach based on specific needs to achieve optimal results and promote overall well-being.

CHAPTER 10: WALL PILATES FOR PROPER POSTURE

Wall Pilates is a highly effective approach to improving and maintaining correct posture. This type of exercise utilizes the support of the wall to emphasize the fundamental elements of Pilates, providing a range of benefits targeted at posture correction. Here's a detailed explanation of the topic:

Fundamental Pilates Principles Applied to the Wall

Core Control: Wall Pilates focuses on core control through exercises engaging deep abdominal muscles, helping stabilize the spine and enhance posture.

Spinal Alignment: Wall exercises promote proper alignment of the spine, reducing pressure on the neck and back and alleviating any muscle tensions.

Release of Tensions: Leveraging the support of the wall allows a focus on releasing muscle tensions and improving flexibility, essential elements for balanced posture.

Specific Benefits of Wall Pilates for Posture

Postural Awareness: Wall Pilates exercises demand increased postural awareness, encouraging individuals to be mindful and correct any incorrect postural habits.

Strength in Postural Muscles: Training against the wall develops strength in postural muscles, such as those in the back, shoulders, and core, essential for supporting an upright posture.

Improved Flexibility: Wall Pilates emphasizes enhanced flexibility, aiding in reducing muscle stiffness that can impact posture.

Examples of Wall Pilates Exercises for Posture

"Wall Angels": Lean against the wall and, keeping the spine against it, perform arm movements resembling an angel, promoting chest openness.

"Spine Stretch": Sitting with the back against the wall, extend the arms upward, creating an elongated line from the top of the head to the sacrum to improve spinal alignment.

"Wall Squats": Perform squats with the back against the wall to strengthen the legs and enhance posture.

Integration into Overall Pilates Routine

Preparation for Complex Exercises: Wall Pilates can serve as preparation for more advanced exercises, ensuring a solid foundation of strength and correct posture.

Customization of the Routine: Adaptable to various needs, Wall Pilates can be customized to address specific postural issues and contribute to achieving individual goals.

Wall Pilates for correct posture emerges as an integrated and targeted approach, providing the necessary tools to correct improper habits and promote healthy and sustainable posture over time.

CHAPTER 11: SPECIFIC EXERCISES FOR BACK WELL-BEING

Specific exercises for back wellness are essential for promoting the health and flexibility of the spine, as well as alleviating any tension or discomfort. These targeted exercises are designed to strengthen the muscles of the back, improve spinal alignment, and enhance mobility. Here's a detailed explanation of the topic:

Objectives of Back Wellness Exercises:

Muscular Strengthening: The exercises are designed to strengthen the muscles of the back, including those in the lumbar, thoracic, and cervical regions.

Improvement of Spinal Alignment: They promote proper spinal alignment, reducing pressure on discs and joints and preventing potential postural issues.

Increase in Flexibility: Specific exercises encourage spinal flexibility, helping to reduce muscle stiffness and improve overall mobility.

Examples of Back Wellness Exercises:

"Cat-Cow Stretch": This yoga exercise involves alternating between arching and rounding the back, contributing to improved flexibility and alignment.

Seated Torso Rotations: While sitting with a straight back, perform torso rotations to work on spinal mobility.

"Child's Pose": A yoga relaxation position that stretches the back, lengthening the spine, and relieving muscle tension.

Core Stabilization Exercises: Movements like leg raises or planks, focusing on core stabilization, help support the back.

Integration with Pilates:

Pilates Bridge: Strengthens the muscles of the back and glutes, improving spinal alignment.

Pilates Roll-Up: Enhances spinal flexibility and strengthens abdominal and paravertebral muscles.

Important Tips:

Medical Consultation: Before starting a new exercise program, it is advisable to consult with a medical professional, especially if there are concerns about back health.

Listening to Your Body: During exercises, it is crucial to listen to your body and avoid movements that cause pain or discomfort.

Specific exercises for back wellness are a valuable component of a comprehensive fitness program, contributing not only to muscle strengthening but also to maintaining a healthy and flexible spine in the long run.

CHAPTER 12: WALL PILATES DURING PREGNANCY

Practicing wall Pilates during pregnancy can offer a range of benefits for expectant mothers, contributing to overall well-being and maintaining appropriate physical fitness. However, it is crucial to adapt exercises to address the specific needs of pregnancy. Here is a detailed explanation of the topic:

Benefits of Wall Pilates During Pregnancy:

Core Stabilization: Wall Pilates exercises can focus on core stabilization, helping to maintain strength in the abdominal area, which is crucial during pregnancy.

Posture Improvement: Promotes correct posture, alleviating any discomfort related to changes in weight distribution.

Back Strengthening: Specific exercises can target the strengthening of back muscles, helping to prevent or alleviate common backaches during pregnancy.

Flexibility and Relaxation: Targeted movements can promote muscle flexibility and relaxation, offering relief from potential tensions.

Adaptations for Pregnancy:

Medical Consultation: Before starting any wall Pilates program during pregnancy, obtaining approval from a doctor is essential.

Attention to Positions: Avoid prolonged supine positions after the first trimester and reduce exercises on the stomach. Also, avoid movements that may cause excessive strain.

Exercise Modifications: Adapt exercises based on body changes. Reduce the range of movements and use supports like pillows or fitness balls, if necessary.

Examples of Wall Pilates Exercises During Pregnancy:

"Wall Squats": Gentle squats with the back against the wall to strengthen the legs and glutes.

Breathing Exercises: Practice deep and controlled breathing, contributing to stress management and overall well-being.

Modified "Leg Lifts": Controlled leg lifts adapted to maintain stability and engage abdominal muscles.

Important Considerations:

Listening to Your Body: Respect the body's signals and stop exercises if you experience pain or discomfort.

Individual Variability: Every pregnancy is unique, so needs and limitations may vary. Adjust the workout accordingly.

Prenatal Pilates Experts: Consider attending prenatal Pilates classes or consulting with an instructor experienced in prenatal practice.

Wall Pilates during pregnancy can be a safe and effective way to maintain physical activity, promoting physical and mental well-being during this special time in a woman's life.

CHAPTER 13: NUTRITIONAL TIPS TO MAXIMIZE RESULTS

Adopting proper nutrition is crucial to maximize the results of any workout program, including Wall Pilates. A balanced diet can contribute to sustaining energy, promoting muscle repair, and improving overall health. Below, I explain in detail the topic of nutritional tips:

Adequate Nutritional Balance: Ensure you get a variety of essential nutrients, including carbohydrates, proteins, healthy fats, vitamins, and minerals. Proper nutritional balance supports body functions and the energy needed for workouts.

Hydration: Maintaining adequate hydration is crucial for the proper functioning of the body. Drinking enough water contributes to joint health, regulates body temperature, and enhances overall performance.

Protein Intake: Proteins are essential for muscle repair and growth. Incorporating sources of lean protein such as chicken, fish, legumes, and dairy can help support the body during training and muscle regeneration.

Complex Carbohydrates: Complex carbohydrates provide a sustainable source of energy. Choose whole grains, fruits, vegetables, and legumes to ensure a consistent intake of carbohydrates throughout the day.

Healthy Fats: Integrate healthy fats found in avocados, nuts, seeds, and olive oil. Healthy fats are important for heart health and provide energy during physical activity.

Meal Planning: Planning regular meals and snacks helps maintain stable energy levels. Avoid skipping meals to prevent energy dips and stimulate metabolism.

Portion Moderation: Controlling portion sizes is crucial. Consuming balanced portions helps avoid excess calories and maintains weight control.

Post-Workout Integration: After a workout, consume a meal or snack containing proteins and carbohydrates to promote muscle repair and energy recovery.

Listening to Your Body: Paying attention to the body's signals is essential. Eating when hungry and stopping when satisfied is an effective way to maintain proper nutritional balance.

Consultation with a Nutritionist: In case of doubts or specific needs, consult a nutritionist or a professional in the field to develop a personalized meal plan.

Following proper nutritional advice is crucial to getting the most out of your Wall Pilates workouts, supporting your overall health, and maximizing desired results.

CHAPTER 14: WEEKLY WORKOUT PLANS FOR DIFFERENT SKILL LEVELS

Welcome to the exploration of weekly workout plans suitable for different skill levels in the context of Wall Pilates. The diversity of skills and physical needs among individuals is a crucial element in designing effective training programs. In this context, weekly workout plans become a fundamental tool for personalizing the training experience, tailoring it to individual abilities, goals, and fitness levels.

This approach aims to provide an accessible and progressive path, allowing anyone, regardless of their level of experience, to fully benefit from Wall Pilates exercises. We will explore weekly routines that cater to beginners, intermediates, and advanced practitioners, carefully designed to provide an optimal balance of strength, flexibility, and body control.

Whether you are starting your Pilates journey or already an experienced practitioner, these weekly workout plans are crafted to accompany you on a journey of continuous improvement. Together, we will discover how to tailor exercises to your needs, always keeping the focus on the fundamental principles of Pilates. Are you ready to explore and customize your workout journey? Let's embark on this path towards lasting physical health and well-being.

Example of Weekly Wall Pilates Workout Plans for Beginners

Week 1: Introduction to Pilates Fundamentals

Day 1:

Light Warm-up: Gentle marching in place (5 minutes)

Wall Exercise: Wall Squats (3 sets of 10 repetitions)

Cool Down: Leg stretching

Day 3:

Warm-up: Shoulder and neck rotations (5 minutes)

Wall Exercise: Wall Push-ups (3 sets of 12 repetitions)

Matwork Exercises: Pilates Matwork for beginners

Cool Down: Trunk stretching

Day 5:

Warm-up: Hip rotations (5 minutes)

Wall Exercise: Modified Leg Lifts (3 sets of 10 repetitions per leg)

Cool Down: Arm and leg stretching

Week 2: Delving into the Principles of Control

Day 1:

Warm-up: Wrist and ankle circles (5 minutes)

Wall Exercise: Wall Plank (3 sets of 30 seconds)

Matwork Exercises: Pilates Matwork emphasizes control

Cool Down: Full-body stretching

Day 3:

Warm-up: Light jogging with knee lifts (5 minutes)

Wall Exercise: Wall Roll-Downs (3 sets of 8 repetitions)

Cool Down: Spine stretching

Day 5:

Warm-up: Twisting torso with side bends (5 minutes)

Wall Exercise: Wall Bridge (3 sets of 12 repetitions)

Cool Down: Hip stretching

Week 3: Consolidation and Progression

Day 1:

Warm-up: Light hopping with knee lifts (5 minutes)

Wall Exercise: Wall Squats with Ball (3 sets of 12 repetitions)

Matwork Exercises: Pilates Matwork with emphasis on control

Cool Down: Full-body stretching

Day 3:

Warm-up: Hip lifts with torso twists (5 minutes)

Wall Exercise: Modified Leg Circles (3 sets of 10 repetitions per direction)

Cool Down: Leg and hip stretching

Day 5:

Warm-up: Side leg lifts (5 minutes)

Wall Exercise: Wall Teaser (3 sets of 8 repetitions)

Cool Down: Torso and shoulder stretching

These weekly programs for beginners are designed to gradually introduce participants to Wall Pilates, focusing on fundamentals and reinforcing body control. Adapt exercises based on your needs and progress gradually. Always consult a health professional before starting a new workout program.

Weekly Wall Pilates Workout Plans for Intermediate-Level

Week 1: Consolidation of Fundamentals and Progression

Day 1:

Warm-up: Jumping jacks and shoulder rotations (5 min)

Wall Exercise: Wall Squats with Ball (4 sets of 12 repetitions)

Matwork Exercises: Intermediate Matwork with a focus on the core

Cool Down: Full-body stretching

Day 3:

Warm-up: Light jogging in place with knee lifts (5 min)

Wall Exercise: Wall Plank with Rotation (4 sets of 20 seconds per side)

Matwork Exercises: Pilates Matwork with emphasis on stability

Cool Down: Trunk and shoulder stretching

Day 5:

Warm-up: Skipping with lateral leg lifts (5 min)

Wall Exercise: Advanced Wall Roll-Downs (4 sets of 10 repetitions)

Matwork Exercises: Advanced Matwork with a focus on control

Cool Down: Leg and hip stretching

Week 2: Strengthening and Flexibility Enhancement

Day 1:

Warm-up: Jump squats and torso rotations (5 min)

Wall Exercise: Wall Teaser with Ball (4 sets of 10 repetitions)

Matwork Exercises: Pilates Matwork with a focus on smooth movements

Cool Down: Full-body stretching

Day 3:

Warm-up: High knees with arm push-ups (5 min)

Wall Exercise: Wall Bridge with Bent Legs (4 sets of 15 repetitions)

Matwork Exercises: Advanced Pilates Matwork focusing on strength

Cool Down: Spine stretching

Day 5:

Warm-up: Running in place with lateral jumps (5 min)

Wall Exercise: Wall Scissor Kicks (4 sets of 12 repetitions per leg)

Matwork Exercises: Pilates Matwork with balance exercises

Cool Down: Arm and shoulder stretching

Week 3: Advancement and Coordination

Day 1:

Warm-up: Burpees and wrist rotations (5 min)

Wall Exercise: Wall Corkscrew (4 sets of 8 repetitions per direction)

Matwork Exercises: Advanced Pilates Matwork with a focus on coordination

Cool Down: Full-body stretching

Day 3:

Warm-up: Running with changes in direction (5 min)

Wall Exercise: Wall Scissor Twist (4 sets of 15 repetitions)

Matwork Exercises: Advanced Pilates Matwork with dynamic exercises

Cool Down: Leg and back stretching

Day 5:

Warm-up: Jump lunges and lateral arm lifts (5 min)

Wall Exercise: Wall Swan Dive (4 sets of 10 repetitions)

Matwork Exercises: Advanced Pilates Matwork with a focus on core strength

Cool Down: Full-body stretching

These weekly programs for the intermediate level aim to consolidate and enhance Wall Pilates fundamentals, introducing more advanced and challenging exercises. Adjust the intensity based on your needs and always consult a healthcare professional before starting a new workout program.

Weekly Wall Pilates Workout Plans for Advanced Level

Week 1: Advanced Core Strengthening

Day 1:

Warm-up: Dynamic stretching and joint rotations (8 min)

Wall Exercise: Wall Pike with Ball (4 sets of 12 repetitions)

Matwork Exercises: Advanced Pilates Matwork focusing on core activation

Cool Down: Full-body stretching

Day 3:

Warm-up: High-intensity interval training (HIIT) cardio (8 min)

Wall Exercise: Wall Handstand Push-ups (4 sets of 10 reps)

Matwork Exercises: Challenging Matwork variations for core strength

Cool Down: Spine and hip flexibility exercises

Day 5:

Warm-up: Plyometric exercises and agility drills (8 min)

Wall Exercise: Wall Plank with Leg Lifts (4 sets of 15 reps per leg)

Matwork Exercises: Pilates advanced routines with twists and advanced bends

Cool Down: Advanced stretching routine targeting major muscle groups

Week 2: Advanced Flexibility and Balance

Day 1:

Warm-up: Cardio Circuit sequences (8 min)

Wall Exercise: Wall Split Stretches (4 sets, holding for 20 seconds each)

Matwork Exercises: Yoga-inspired Pilates Matwork for flexibility

Cool Down: Lengthening stretches for muscles and joints

Day 3:

Warm-up: Cardio Circuit sequences (8 min)

Wall Exercise: Wall Arabesque (4 sets of 12 reps per leg)

Matwork Exercises: Controlled Pilates movements for enhanced balance

Cool Down: Deep stretches emphasizing balance and flexibility

Day 5:

Warm-up: Ballet-inspired dynamic stretches (8 min)

Wall Exercise: Wall Side Plank with Leg Raise (4 sets of 15 reps per side)

Matwork Exercises: Flowing Pilates routine with emphasis on balance

Cool Down: Graceful stretches promoting flexibility

Week 3: Advanced Full-Body Integration

Day 1:

Warm-up: Cardio circuit incorporating bodyweight exercises (8 min)

Wall Exercise: Wall Spiderman Push-ups (4 sets of 12 reps)

Matwork Exercises: Full-body Pilates routine with advanced variations

Cool Down: Comprehensive stretching routine for muscles and joints

Day 3:

Warm-up: Kettlebell-inspired dynamic movements (8 min)

Wall Exercise: Wall Roll-Downs with Ball (4 sets of 10 reps)

Matwork Exercises: Dynamic Pilates routine for overall strength and flexibility

Cool Down: Targeted stretches for muscle recovery

Day 5:

Warm-up: High-intensity interval training (HIIT) with a focus on explosive power (8 min)

Wall Exercise: Wall Lateral Jumps (4 sets of 15 reps)

Matwork Exercises: Integrative Pilates routine incorporating advanced elements

Cool Down: Relaxing stretching for enhanced flexibility and mental focus

These weekly programs for advanced practitioners aim to challenge and enhance core strength, flexibility, and balance. Adjust the intensity based on your capabilities and consult with a healthcare professional before starting a new advanced workout program.

CHAPTER 15: INCORPORATING WALL PILATES INTO DAILY LIFE

In the realm of fitness, the benefits of Pilates extend beyond the confines of a workout space, allowing individuals to seamlessly integrate its principles into their daily lives. Incorporating Wall Pilates into your routine provides an opportunity to enhance physical well-being, promote mindfulness, and foster a balanced lifestyle.

Mindful Movement in Daily Activities: One key aspect of integrating Wall Pilates into daily life is the application of mindful movement. By being conscious of posture, alignment, and controlled breathing during routine activities like sitting at a desk, walking, or lifting objects, individuals can cultivate a heightened awareness of their body's movements. This mindfulness not only supports the principles of Pilates but also contributes to better posture and reduced strain on muscles.

Functional Core Engagement: The core is at the center of Pilates, and incorporating its principles into daily activities helps in maintaining a strong and engaged core. Whether standing in line, waiting for an elevator, or even washing dishes, the conscious engagement of the core muscles enhances stability and supports the spine, promoting a more functional and resilient body.

Quick Wall Pilates Breaks: Incorporating short Wall Pilates routines into breaks throughout the day is another effective strategy. Simple wall exercises, such as Wall Squats or Wall Planks, can be seamlessly integrated into daily routines. These quick breaks not only contribute to physical fitness but also serve as rejuvenating mental pauses, helping individuals return to tasks with increased focus and energy.

Mind-Body Connection: The mind-body connection emphasized in Pilates extends beyond the studio walls. Translating this connection into daily life involves being present in the moment, listening to the body's signals, and making conscious choices to move with intention. This holistic approach contributes to a sense of well-being and can positively impact overall mental and emotional health.

Efficient Use of Time: One of the advantages of incorporating Wall Pilates into daily life is its efficiency. Short, targeted exercises can be seamlessly woven into busy schedules, making them more accessible for individuals with hectic lifestyles. This efficient use of time makes it easier to prioritize physical well-being without requiring a dedicated workout session.

In summary, incorporating Wall Pilates into everyday life goes beyond the physical aspects of exercise. It becomes a holistic approach to movement, posture, and mindfulness. By integrating Pilates principles into routine activities, individuals can experience the transformative benefits of Pilates throughout their day, promoting not just physical fitness but a more balanced and mindful lifestyle.

In addition to the mentioned benefits, integrating Wall Pilates into daily life offers a range of advantages that contribute to long-term physical and mental well-being. Here are further positive aspects of this practice within the scope of daily activities:

Stress and Tension Reduction: Incorporating Wall Pilates exercises during breaks throughout the day can act as a form of active relaxation. Controlled movements, mindful breathing, and stretching contribute to reducing accumulated stress and muscle tension, promoting an overall sense of calm and well-being.

Posture Improvement: Posture awareness during daily activities is a key element of Pilates. Integrating these principles helps correct poor posture and prevent back pain associated with misalignment. Proper posture not only reduces the risk of musculoskeletal issues but also contributes to a more confident and secure appearance.

Boost in Energy and Vitality: Even short sessions of Wall Pilates can act as a stimulating "recharge" during the day. Movements involving the entire body, even if brief, increase blood circulation and enhance energy flow, providing a sense of vitality and renewed focus.

Heightened Body Awareness: Practicing Wall Pilates allows for a deeper connection with one's body. Awareness of movements, alignment, and breathing translates into greater body awareness, leading to more conscious choices regarding nutrition, rest, and stress management.

Metabolism Boost and Muscle Tone: Activating the core and other muscle groups during Wall Pilates exercises contributes to boosting metabolism and improving muscle tone. This not only aids in achieving a leaner physique but also supports the overall health of the musculoskeletal system.

Sleep Improvement: Regular exercise, even if brief, is linked to improvements in sleep quality. Integrating Wall Pilates into your daily routine can contribute to reducing insomnia, enhancing sleep quality, and promoting more rejuvenating rest.

Flexibility and Joint Mobility: Wall Pilates exercises are designed to improve flexibility and joint mobility. Maintaining flexible muscles and joints contributes not only to injury prevention but also facilitates daily movement, making it more agile and efficient.

Integrating Wall Pilates into your daily life offers a holistic approach to well-being, contributing not only to your physical fitness but also to your mental balance and overall quality of life.

CHAPTER 16: ADDRESSING COMMON CONCERNS AND QUESTIONS

The introduction of Wall Pilates into your routine may raise common questions and concerns. Let's address some of the most frequently asked questions and provide answers to alleviate any doubts.

1. "Can I practice Wall Pilates even if I'm a beginner?"

Absolutely yes. Wall Pilates workouts can be adapted to various skill levels. There are exercises specifically designed for beginners that allow you to gradually build strength and flexibility. Start with basic exercises and progressively increase the intensity as you gain confidence.

2. "What are the specific benefits of Wall Pilates compared to other forms of Pilates?"

Wall Pilates offers additional support and a variety of exercise options that can intensify your workout. The use of the wall can improve stability and allow for a greater range of motion in certain positions. Additionally, the wall can serve as a visual guide to ensure proper exercise execution.

3. "Can I practice Wall Pilates at home?"

Absolutely yes. Many Wall Pilates routines are designed to be conveniently performed at home. You just need an open space near a wall. You can follow step-by-step instructions to ensure that exercises are performed correctly.

4. "Does Wall Pilates require special equipment?"

Typically, no special equipment is required. However, you may want to use a yoga mat for comfort during floor exercises. Some exercises may involve the use of a Pilates ball or other small props, but often they can be adapted without them.

5. "Are there any contraindications for Wall Pilates?"

For most people, Wall Pilates is safe and beneficial. However, if you have health issues or specific concerns, it's advisable to consult a healthcare professional before starting a new exercise program. Additionally, always listen to your body and modify exercises based on your needs.

6. "How much time should I dedicate to Wall Pilates to see results?"

The frequency and duration depend on your individual needs and goals. Even a few sessions per week can lead to improvements. Consistency is key. Start with shorter sessions and gradually increase the duration as your strength and endurance improve.

7. "Can I combine Wall Pilates with other forms of exercise?"

Certainly. Wall Pilates can be effectively integrated with other forms of exercise, such as cardio or weight training. Variety can be beneficial for your overall routine and offer complementary benefits.

8. "Can I practice Wall Pilates if I have back issues?"

Wall Pilates can be adapted to fit many physical conditions, but it's advisable to consult with a healthcare professional before starting, especially if you have back issues. Some exercises may need to be modified or avoided depending on your situation.

9. "How can I adapt exercises if I have limited space?"

If space is limited, you can select exercises that require smaller movements or adjust the body's angle to fit the available space. It's important to perform exercises safely, avoiding objects or walls that could cause injury.

10. "What is suitable attire for practicing Wall Pilates?"

The attire should be comfortable, allow a full range of movement, and not cause skin irritations. It's advisable to wear fitted but not overly tight clothing. Gym shoes are usually not necessary as many exercises are performed barefoot or with non-slip socks.

11. "Can I practice Wall Pilates during pregnancy?"

Practicing Wall Pilates during pregnancy can be safe, but it's essential to consult with your doctor and preferably work with a Pilates instructor specializing in pregnancy. Modifications to exercises will be necessary to accommodate the needs of the growing body and ensure safety.

12. "How long does it take to master advanced exercises?"

The time needed to master advanced exercises varies from person to person. Consistent practice, proper execution, and attention to form are crucial. Start with basic exercises and progress gradually as you develop strength and control.

13. "Can I practice Wall Pilates with specific health conditions, such as high blood pressure?"

It's important to consult with your doctor before starting any exercise program, especially if you have specific health conditions such as hypertension. Wall Pilates can be adapted, but some positions may need to be modified or avoided.

14. "Are there specific exercises to improve flexibility?"

Yes, there are Wall Pilates exercises specifically designed to improve flexibility. These often involve positions that utilize the support of the wall to facilitate relaxation and muscle stretching.

Remember that these answers are general and may vary based on individual circumstances. Always consult with a healthcare professional or a Pilates instructor for personalized advice based on your physical condition.

CHAPTER 17: PSYCHOLOGICAL ASPECTS OF EXERCISE: MOTIVATION AND CONSISTENCY

Physical exercise is not merely an act of physical commitment but deeply involves the psychological aspect of the individual engaging in it. In the following chapter, we will explore the intricate aspects of motivation and consistency within the realm of physical exercise, with a particular focus on the context of Wall Pilates.

Motivation, often the initial spark that ignites the flame of physical activity, is a crucial element in sustaining an active lifestyle. We will delve into the different sources of motivation and how we can nurture them to support consistent commitment over time. From discovering personal goals to the influence of the surrounding environment, we will explore the psychological levers that can fuel our willingness to pursue health through Wall Pilates.

Consistency, the steadfast companion of motivation, plays a fundamental role in transforming isolated efforts into genuine habits. We will examine common challenges that threaten consistency and provide practical strategies to overcome them. Through the analysis of workout routines, realistic goal-setting, and stress management techniques, we will explore how to maintain a steadfast commitment to both physical and mental well-being.

A holistic approach to these psychological aspects of exercise is essential to creating a strong and sustainable foundation for our health journey. Through this exploration, our aim is not only to provide a comprehensive understanding of the psychological mechanisms but also practical tools to cultivate enduring motivation and consistency that will lead to lasting results in our Wall Pilates journey and beyond.

Motivation in the Context of Wall Pilates

Motivation in the context of Wall Pilates plays a crucial role in sustaining consistent commitment and maximizing the physical and mental benefits of this practice. Let's take a closer look at how motivation can positively impact your journey with Wall Pilates:

Discovering Personal Goals. The key to lasting motivation in Wall Pilates is the discovery and clear definition of personal goals. These goals can be related to health, physical well-being, flexibility, or acquiring new skills. Having a clear goal provides a tangible purpose, fueling intrinsic motivation.

Creating a Fulfilling Routine. A Wall Pilates routine that fits your lifestyle and is personally fulfilling can significantly contribute to motivation. Experimenting with different exercise sequences, discovering those you enjoy the most, and adapting the practice to your preferences can make the workout more rewarding, keeping motivation alive in the long run.

Cultivating a Positive Mindset. Maintaining a positive mindset is crucial for continuous motivation. Celebrating progress, even small achievements, and focusing on the positive aspects of the practice contribute to creating a cycle of reward that fuels the desire to continue.

Social Engagement. Sharing your Wall Pilates experience with others can add a social component that strengthens motivation. A workout partner or participating in group classes can create a supportive environment, making exercise more enjoyable and engaging.

Adaptation and Variation. Motivation can wane if the workout becomes monotonous. Introducing variations into your routine, trying new exercises, or incorporating periodic challenges can keep the enthusiasm alive. Variety stimulates the mind and body, preventing fatigue and a decline in motivation.

Reflecting on Benefits. Reflecting on the benefits derived from regular Wall Pilates practice can reinforce motivation. Whether it's physical improvements, stress reduction, or an overall enhancement of well-being, taking time to appreciate the results achieved can fuel the determination to continue.

In summary, motivation in the context of Wall Pilates is a powerful engine for maintaining a consistent and fulfilling practice. By leveraging personal goals, enjoyable routines, a positive mindset, social engagement, workout variation, and reflecting on the benefits, you can cultivate lasting motivation that supports your journey to physical and mental well-being.

Consistency in the Context of Wall Pilates

Consistency in the context of Wall Pilates is a key element to maximize the benefits of the practice and achieve tangible results over time. Let's take a closer look at how consistency can positively impact your journey with Wall Pilates:

Regular Workout Routine. Consistency implies regular practice over time. Establishing a workout routine that incorporates Wall Pilates into your daily life helps build healthy habits. Scheduling regular sessions contributes to maintaining a consistent presence in your life, creating a solid foundation for well-being.

Realistic Goals and Gradual Progression. Setting realistic and progressively challenging goals is essential for maintaining consistency. Working towards achievable goals provides clear direction, while gradual progression prevents excessive fatigue, keeping long-term interest intact.

Stress Management and Adaptation. Consistency can be undermined by periods of stress or changes in daily life. Learning to manage stress and adapting your Wall Pilates practice based on circumstances maintains flexibility and allows you to continue to engage even during more demanding periods.

Adequate Rest and Recovery. Integral to consistency is recognizing the importance of rest and recovery. Scheduling adequate breaks between workout sessions helps the body recover and prevents the risk of injuries. Smart consistency involves a balanced management of intensity and rest.

Adaptation to Variations. Life is susceptible to variations and unforeseen events. Maintaining consistency doesn't necessarily mean rigidly adhering to a routine in every circumstance, but rather adapting to variations. You can modify exercises based on needs or find alternatives when access to certain equipment is limited.

Self-assessment and Overcoming Obstacles. Consistent practice requires periodic self-assessment. Identifying obstacles or challenges that may undermine consistency and finding solutions to overcome them is crucial. This self-assessment helps you maintain a steadfast commitment to your practice.

In summary, consistency in the context of Wall Pilates is a key element to experiencing the maximum benefits of the practice in the long run. Developing a routine, setting realistic goals, managing stress, adapting to variations, and periodically self-assessing are all fundamental elements to maintain a Wall Pilates practice that contributes to your physical and mental well-being.

CHAPTER 18: PROGRESS OVER TIME: HOW TO MEASURE AND MONITOR

Measuring and monitoring progress over time is an essential aspect of your journey with Wall Pilates. This process not only provides tangible feedback on your results but can also be a source of continuous motivation. Let's explore how you can measure and monitor your progress over time:

Progress Journal. Maintaining a progress journal is an effective method. It can include information such as the type of exercises, the number of repetitions, the duration of sessions, and any particular feelings or personal notes. This journal becomes a reference framework that allows you to look back and assess improvements over time.

Periodic Physical Assessment. Scheduling regular physical assessments is a formal way to measure progress. These assessments may include body measurements, flexibility tests, muscle strength, and other relevant metrics. Comparisons between periodic assessments offer a clear view of physical developments.

Before and After Photographs. Taking before and after photographs can be a visual way to monitor progress. Images can highlight changes in posture, muscle tone, or body composition. Even if changes are subtle, photographs provide a tangible representation of the results achieved.

Sensations and Overall Well-being. In addition to objective measurements, taking note of sensations and overall well-being is equally important. You might notice improvements in sleep quality, energy levels, or stress management. These signals indicate benefits beyond physical measurements.

Achieving Specific Goals. Setting specific and measurable goals gives you a clear compass to measure progress. These goals could be related to improvements in flexibility, mastering more advanced exercises, or reaching specific levels of endurance. Achieving these goals serves as a tangible indicator of your success.

Instructor or Workout Partner Feedback. Getting feedback from a qualified instructor or a workout partner can provide an external and objective perspective on your progress. These individuals may notice improvements in technique, posture, or endurance that you might not immediately perceive.

In summary, measuring and monitoring progress over time in the context of Wall Pilates is a holistic approach that embraces both objective data and subjective feelings. This process not only provides a clear insight into your physical improvements but also serves as a continuous source of motivation to pursue your wellness journey with commitment and confidence.

Setting Specific Goals in the Context of Wall Pilates

In the context of Wall Pilates, you can set a range of specific goals that align with the benefits you aim to derive from this practice. Here are some examples of specific goals you might consider:

Improving Flexibility.

 Goal: Achieve a specific increase in degrees of flexibility in certain areas of the body, such as the spine or leg joints, within a predetermined timeframe.

Muscle Strengthening.

Goal: Increase muscle strength, for example, in core muscles, legs, or arms, by measuring increased resistance or the ability to complete more advanced exercises.

Posture Correction.

Goal: Improve posture through specific exercises, working on specific muscles that influence proper body alignment. Measure improvements through photos or body awareness.

Mastery of Advanced Exercises.

Goal: Attain the ability to perform more advanced and complex exercises in the context of Wall Pilates, demonstrating increased technical proficiency and muscle control.

Increased Cardiovascular Endurance.

Goal: Integrate Wall Pilates elements that promote an increase in cardiovascular endurance, measuring improvement in the ability to sustain dynamic and prolonged exercises.

Stress Reduction and Mental Well-being Improvement.
Goal: Use Wall Pilates as a tool to reduce stress and enhance mental well-being. Monitor stress levels and overall well-being over time.

Consistency in Practice.

Goal: Establish a regular Wall Pilates routine, committing to practice consistently and recording the frequency of weekly sessions.

Improvement in Coordination and Balance.

Goal: Focus on targeted exercises that enhance coordination and balance, measuring stability and confidence in movements over time.

Sleep Quality Improvement. Goal:

Use Wall Pilates to improve sleep quality. Measure sleep duration and quality over time.

Reduction of Pain or Muscle Tension.

Goal: Use specific exercises to reduce pain or muscle tension in specific areas of the body. Monitor improvements through self-assessments or medical consultation.

Customize these goals based on your needs and the specific objectives you want to achieve with Wall Pilates. Ensure you set realistic, measurable goals with a defined time frame to maintain your motivation and track your progress.

CHAPTER 19: WALL PILATES FOR WOMEN: DETAILED INSIGHTS

Wall Pilates represents an effective and versatile way to engage in physical exercise, particularly well-suited for women. This integrative practice combines Pilates principles with the use of a wall for support, offering specific advantages for women's well-being. Here are detailed insights regarding the context of Wall Pilates for women:

Core Strength Focus:

Wall Pilates places a strong emphasis on core strengthening, including the abdominal, lumbar, and pelvic muscles. This is particularly significant for women as it helps improve trunk stability, supports posture, and can be beneficial during pregnancy.

Hormonal Balance:

Women often experience hormonal variations during different life phases such as puberty, pregnancy, and menopause. Wall Pilates, with its targeted approach to body and mind control, can help manage these hormonal changes by reducing stress and enhancing overall well-being.

Posture and Flexibility:

Women are susceptible to postural changes, especially due to factors like wearing high heels and a sedentary lifestyle. Wall Pilates can contribute to correcting posture through specific exercises, simultaneously improving flexibility and reducing muscle tension.

Weight Management and Muscle Tone:

Wall Pilates can be an effective component of a weight management program, involving the entire body and promoting muscle tone. By integrating targeted cardiovascular exercises, it can contribute to maintaining a healthy weight and achieving fitness goals.

Pelvic Health:

Pelvic health is a significant concern for many women. Wall Pilates can offer benefits for pelvic floor health through specific exercises that work on awareness and control of pelvic muscles, contributing to the prevention of issues like incontinence.

Injury Prevention:

Women are at risk for some specific injuries, such as those related to intense physical activity or improper movements. Wall Pilates, with its controlled and targeted approach, can contribute to injury prevention by improving strength, flexibility, and body awareness.

Emotional Wellness:

Wall Pilates is also an opportunity to promote emotional well-being. The practice emphasizes the mind-body connection, encouraging breath awareness, and reducing stress. This can be particularly relevant for women who often manage multiple responsibilities.

Adaptability to Pregnancy:

During pregnancy, Wall Pilates can be adapted to meet the specific needs of pregnant women. It provides a safe method to maintain strength and flexibility, contributing to physical well-being during this phase of life.

Body Awareness:

The practice of Wall Pilates encourages body awareness, helping women develop a greater awareness of movements and physical sensations. This can be particularly useful for improving posture, reducing muscle tension, and preventing injuries.

Socialization and Support:

Participating in Wall Pilates classes can offer women a social and supportive environment. Sharing the experience with other women can enhance motivation, accountability, and the creation of a support network.

Stress Management and Mental Health:

Wall Pilates can be a valuable ally in stress management. Through targeted exercises and a focus on breathing, it can contribute to reducing stress levels and improving the mental health of women.

Pelvic Floor Strengthening:

One of the distinctive advantages for women is the strengthening of the pelvic floor. Specific Wall Pilates exercises can promote muscle tone in this area, helping to prevent or alleviate issues related to pelvic floor health.

Sustainability and Adaptability:

Wall Pilates is a sustainable approach that can be adapted to different fitness levels and personal goals. Its versatility makes it accessible to women of all ages and physical conditions.

Joint Strengthening:

By focusing on the proper execution of movements and alignment, Wall Pilates can contribute to joint strengthening, providing a particular benefit for women who may be more susceptible to joint problems.

Holistic Approach to Health:

Wall Pilates goes beyond the physical aspect and embraces a holistic approach to health. Integrating elements of mindfulness and awareness can contribute to enhancing the overall well-being of body and mind.

Flexibility and Convenience:

This practice offers flexibility in timing, allowing women to easily integrate Wall Pilates into their daily routine. The option to exercise at home makes this form of training extremely convenient.

Improvement of Blood Circulation:

Pilates exercises, including those performed at the wall, can promote blood circulation. This is particularly relevant for women, contributing to maintaining cardiovascular health and strengthening the circulatory system.

Postural Awareness in Daily Life:

Teachings from Wall Pilates can transfer into daily life, increasing postural awareness during activities such as sitting at work and improving body alignment in various situations.

Motivation Through Exercise Variety:

The diversity of exercises offered by Wall Pilates can keep women motivated, providing a variety of movements that stimulate both the body and the mind.

Promotion of Self-Esteem:

Improving strength, flexibility, and body awareness through Wall Pilates can contribute to promoting self-esteem in women, providing a sense of personal achievement and well-being.

These insights highlight the wealth of benefits that Wall Pilates can offer women, going beyond the physical aspect to embrace a comprehensive perspective on health and well-being.

CHAPTER 20: KEY POINTS OF THE BOOK

Introduction:

Presentation of the concept of Wall Pilates.

Contextualization of the specific approach tailored for women.

Pilates Fundamentals: Basic Principles:

Detailed explanation of the fundamental principles of Pilates.

In-depth exploration of Control, Center, Flow of Movement, Precision, Breathing, and Concentration.

Preparation and Necessary Equipment:

Guide to proper preparation before commencing workouts.

List of necessary equipment for an effective Wall Pilates practice.

Effective Warm-up Before Exercise:

Importance of warming up in the context of Wall Pilates.

Goals of warm-up and examples of targeted exercises.

Wall Pilates Workouts for Beginners:

Introduction to a series of exercises suitable for beginners.

Focus on fundamental principles and a gradual approach.

Focus on Flexibility and Joint Mobility:

Definition of flexibility and joint mobility.

Specific exercises to enhance flexibility through Wall Pilates.

Balance and Coordination in Wall Pilates:

Definition of balance and coordination.

In-depth exploration of the benefits of these aspects in Wall Pilates practice.

Integration of specific exercises to improve dynamic balance.

Wall Pilates Muscle Toning Routine:

Description of a comprehensive routine to tone various muscle groups.

Examples of advanced exercises to stimulate muscle strength.

Weight Management and Cardiovascular Workouts:

In-depth discussion on how Wall Pilates can contribute to weight management.

Integration of cardiovascular exercises and promotion of an active lifestyle.

Wall Pilates for Correct Posture:

Role of Wall Pilates in improving posture.

Specific exercises to promote proper alignment.

Specific Exercises for Back Well-being:

In-depth exploration of how Wall Pilates can benefit back health.

Examples of targeted exercises to alleviate back pain.

Wall Pilates during Pregnancy:

Recommended adaptations for pregnant women.

Benefits of Wall Pilates during this phase.

Nutritional Tips to Maximize Results:

Tips on complementary nutrition alongside Wall Pilates practice.

Weekly Workout Plans for Various Abilities:

Introduction to weekly workout plans for beginners, intermediates, and advanced practitioners.

Incorporating Wall Pilates into Daily Life:

In-depth exploration of integrating Wall Pilates teachings into daily routines.

Additional benefits beyond the physical aspect.

Addressing Common Concerns and Questions:

Response to common questions and solutions to frequently raised concerns.

Providing clarity on specific aspects of the practice.

Psychological Aspects of Exercise: Motivation and Consistency:

Exploration of psychological factors related to regular Wall Pilates practice.

Motivation and consistency as key elements for enduring results.

Progress Over Time: How to Measure and Monitor Results:

Guide on how to measure progress over time.

Importance of monitoring results to maintain motivation.

Specific Goals in the Context of Wall Pilates:

Definition of personalized and specific goals for Wall Pilates practice.

In-Depth Insights Regarding Wall Pilates for Women:

A comprehensive exploration of specific benefits that Wall Pilates offers to women.

CHAPTER 21: CONCLUSION: EMPOWERING WOMEN THROUGH WALL PILATES

In concluding our journey through "Wall Pilates for Women", it's evident that this book is more than just a guide to exercises – it's a holistic approach to wellness tailored specifically for women. We've delved into the intricacies of Pilates, explored the synergy between body and mind, and empowered women to take charge of their physical and mental well-being.

The book begins by introducing the innovative concept of Wall Pilates, setting the stage for a unique and effective fitness journey. Through meticulous guidance on Pilates fundamentals, readers have gained a deep understanding of Control, Centering, Flow of Movement, Precision, Breathing, and Concentration – the pillars of a transformative Pilates practice.

Preparation and equipment discussions ensure that women embark on their Pilates journey equipped with the knowledge and tools necessary for success. The importance of a thorough warm-up, highlighted in the early chapters, lays the foundation for safe and effective workouts.

Tailoring Wall Pilates for beginners has made this discipline accessible to all, emphasizing the gradual incorporation of exercises and principles. Flexibility and joint mobility, crucial elements for overall well-being, are addressed through specialized exercises, allowing women to experience the full spectrum of Pilates benefits.

Balance and coordination, often overlooked aspects of fitness, are elevated in the context of Wall Pilates. The Muscle Toning Routine, meticulously outlined, provides a roadmap to sculpting and strengthening various muscle groups. The book doesn't merely stop at physical exercise; it delves into weight management, cardiovascular workouts, and the intricate relationship between Pilates and a healthy lifestyle.

The emphasis on correct posture and specific exercises for back well-being speaks to the book's commitment to holistic health. For pregnant women, the adaptation of exercises ensures a safe and beneficial Pilates experience during this transformative period.

Nutritional tips add a layer of comprehensive care, recognizing the integral connection between diet and fitness. The inclusion of weekly workout plans caters to varying abilities, promoting inclusivity in the world of Pilates.

As we explore the integration of Pilates into daily life, the book emphasizes that the benefits extend far beyond the physical. It's about fostering mental resilience, empowering women to overcome common concerns, and addressing the psychological aspects of motivation and consistency.

Measuring progress over time becomes an integral part of the journey, reinforcing the idea that every step forward is a victory. Setting specific goals, both personal and physical, provides a roadmap for continual growth and achievement.

The in-depth insights into Wall Pilates for women showcase a commitment to acknowledging and addressing the unique needs and strengths of the female body. It's not just about exercise; it's about empowering women to embrace their bodies, cultivate strength, and embark on a journey of self-discovery.

In the closing pages of "Pilates al Muro per Donne," readers are not bidding farewell to a routine; instead, they are equipped with the tools to perpetuate a lifestyle that intertwines physical and mental well-being. It's an ode to the

strength, resilience, and beauty that every woman possesses –
a celebration of empowerment through Wall Pilates.

In concluding this book, let's add additional layers of
awareness and inspiration to the journey we've undertaken
together. This book is not just an exercise guide; it's an
invitation to explore one's inner strength and celebrate the
diversity of women's experiences.

Wall Pilates is not merely a series of physical movements but
a means through which women can deeply connect with their
bodies. What makes this journey unique is its personalized
approach, recognizing that every woman is an individual with
unique needs and goals.

Beyond physical exercises, the book promotes self-awareness
and acceptance of one's body. It encourages women to
consider Wall Pilates not just as a fitness practice but as an act
of self-love and respect for their bodies.

The section on progress over time and specific goals provides
a clear framework of how the journey in Wall Pilates can
evolve. It emphasizes that success is not only measured in
tangible physical results but also in mental well-being and
self-awareness.

Moreover, the book invites women to explore the concept of
balance in daily life. It highlights that balance is not just about
the ability to stand on one leg but also about balancing
different spheres of life—work, family, mental health, and
self-care.

The section dedicated to weekly workout plans provides a
practical tool to integrate Wall Pilates into daily routines. This
is not just an exercise manual but a resource that can be used
flexibly, adapting to individual needs and the pace of each
woman's life.

Finally, "Pilates al Muro per Donne" celebrates the community of women embracing this journey. It recognizes that the strength of each woman is amplified when shared with others and encourages readers to share their success stories, thereby inspiring more women to embark on their Wall Pilates journey.

In essence, this book is an invitation for all women to discover their strength, embrace their potential, and transform Wall Pilates into a journey of self-determination and personal growth. May this guide be a valuable tool in every woman's path toward complete well-being.

EXTRA CONTENT

Integrating Other Fitness Activities with Wall Pilates

Integrating various fitness activities with Wall Pilates can further enrich the workout experience and provide a more comprehensive perspective on improving health and well-being. Here are some fitness activities that can be seamlessly incorporated with Wall Pilates:

Traditional Strength Exercises: Adding weightlifting exercises or using resistance equipment can further strengthen muscles and improve overall toning. Combining Wall Pilates with traditional strength exercises can provide a comprehensive full-body workout.

Cardiovascular Fitness: Integrating cardiovascular activities like running, swimming, or cycling can improve cardiorespiratory efficiency and promote weight loss. Alternating Wall Pilates with cardio sessions can bring benefits to both strength and cardiovascular health.

Functional Training: Incorporating functional training exercises, involving complex movements similar to those in daily life, can enhance stability and coordination. Using equipment such as medicine balls or resistance bands can add variety and challenge.

Dance: Adding dance classes or choreographed movements can improve movement fluidity and stimulate creativity. This integration may be particularly appealing to those who enjoy a more artistic approach to fitness.

Equipment-Based Pilates: Occasionally integrating Wall Pilates sessions with classes on traditional Pilates equipment, such as the Reformer or Cadillac, can provide a variety of muscle stimuli and a different challenge.

Relaxation Techniques: These are crucial to enhance body awareness, reduce muscle tension, and improve the quality of movement.

The key is to find a balance that suits individual needs and brings physical and mental benefits. Before starting any new fitness program or integrating various activities, it's always advisable to consult with a fitness professional to ensure it aligns with individual physical conditions and goals.

Traditional Strength Exercises in the Context of Wall Pilates for Women

The integration of "Traditional Strength Exercises" in the context of "Wall Pilates for Women" adds a crucial element to the workout program, focusing on increasing muscular strength more conventionally. While Wall Pilates emphasizes core strength, flexibility, and stabilization, traditional strength exercises aim to strengthen specific muscle groups in more traditional ways.

Here are some key points on how "Traditional Strength Exercises" can be effectively integrated:

Specific Muscle Empowerment: While Wall Pilates engages various muscle groups in a more holistic way, traditional strength exercises allow for a more specific focus on certain areas of the body. This can be particularly beneficial for women aiming for specific strength or toning goals.

Use of Weights or Resistance Equipment: Traditional strength exercises often involve the use of free weights, gym machines, or resistance equipment. This can add variety and additional challenge to the workout, enabling women to progressively increase the load and enhance muscular endurance.

Diversification of Muscle Stimuli: Integrating traditional strength exercises can diversify muscle stimuli, leading to greater adaptability and overall strength. This diversification can help prevent workout plateaus, where the body becomes accustomed to certain movements.

Adaptation to Individual Fitness Levels: The beauty of integrating traditional strength exercises is that they can be adapted to individual fitness levels. From beginners to more advanced women, it's possible to customize the training to meet specific needs.

Variety in Muscle Response: While Wall Pilates promotes muscular endurance through the use of body weight, traditional strength exercises offer a different muscle response. This can lead to more noticeable muscle growth, fostering greater definition and toning.

Synergy with Pilates Principles: Integrating traditional strength exercises can synergize with the principles of Wall Pilates, providing a solid foundation of strength to enhance the execution of Pilates movements and further empower the core.

Ultimately, integrating "Traditional Strength Exercises" can be an effective strategy to enrich the workout experience in the context of "Wall Pilates for Women," contributing to a more comprehensive approach to muscular empowerment and overall well-being.

Integrated Training Program: Wall Pilates with Strength Exercises

This training program is designed for women looking to integrate Wall Pilates with traditional strength exercises. The goal is to provide a comprehensive workout, enhancing muscular strength, flexibility, and stability.

Day 1: Core and Abdominals Focus

Wall Pilates:

Core Basics (Plank, Side Plank)

Spinal Flexibility Exercises

Strength Exercises:

Barbell Squats

Dumbbell Lunges

Russian Twists with Weight

Day 2: Arm and Shoulder Empowerment

Wall Pilates:

Shoulder Mobility Exercises

Basic Positions with Emphasis on Arms

Strength Exercises:

Military Press with Dumbbells

Barbell Curls

Lateral Raises with Resistance Band

Day 3: Full-Body Training

Wall Pilates:

Full Movement Flow

Leg Strength Exercises

Strength Exercises:

Barbell Deadlifts

Pull-ups or Lat Pulldowns

Plank Renegade Rows

Day 4: Active Recovery and Stretching

Wall Pilates:

Breathing Exercises and Relaxation

Dynamic Full-Body Stretching

Strength Exercises:

Light mobility exercises and muscle activation

Day 5: Leg and Glute Empowerment

Wall Pilates:

Leg Strengthening Exercises

Basic Positions with Emphasis on Legs

Strength Exercises:

Kettlebell Plié Squats

Side Lunges

Barbell Glute Bridges

Important Note:

Perform each exercise with proper form and controlled breathing.

Adjust the weight and intensity of strength exercises based on your fitness level.

Consult a fitness professional before starting a new training program.

This balanced program offers the versatility of Wall Pilates for core stability and strength, integrated with strength exercises to improve muscular endurance and achieve a complete workout.

Cardio Fitness in the Context of Wall Pilates for Women

In the context of "Wall Pilates for Women," the topic of cardio fitness focuses on integrating exercises aimed at improving cardiovascular health, endurance, and overall physical conditioning. While Wall Pilates is known for emphasizing core strength and flexibility, it's possible to integrate cardiovascular elements to achieve a holistic approach to women's fitness.

Key Points:

Cardio in Wall Pilates:

Introducing more dynamic and rhythmic movements within the framework of Wall Pilates can elevate heart rate and increase blood flow, contributing to cardiovascular effects.

Integrated Cardiovascular Exercises:

Adding exercises such as light jogging, stationary running, or dynamic squats can provide cardiovascular benefits without compromising the fundamental principles of Pilates.

Interval Training:

Incorporating interval training sessions, alternating high-intensity phases with recovery periods, can improve both cardiovascular endurance and muscle toning.

Continuous Flow:

Developing fluid and continuous movement sequences, and maintaining a steady pace, can stimulate the cardiovascular system without sacrificing the control and precision typical of Pilates.

Variety of Movements:

Introducing a variety of multi-planar movements can engage different muscle groups and encourage increased cardiovascular involvement.

Heart Rate Monitoring:

Using heart rate monitoring devices during training ensures that the intensity level achieved contributes to cardiovascular fitness goals.

Adaptation to Fitness Level:

Women of different fitness levels can tailor the intensity of cardiovascular training according to their needs, ensuring a gradual progression.

Combined Benefits:

Integrating cardio fitness into Wall Pilates can lead to combined benefits, including improvements in strength, flexibility, endurance, and overall cardiovascular health.

The integrated approach of cardio fitness in the context of Wall Pilates for women provides a balanced way to achieve comprehensive physical fitness, combining the benefits of Pilates' strength and flexibility with the positive effects of cardiovascular training.

Integrated Training Program: Wall Pilates with Cardio Fitness

This training program is designed for women looking to integrate Wall Pilates exercises with elements of cardio fitness for a comprehensive workout, enhancing strength, flexibility, and cardiovascular health.

Day 1: Balanced Start with Light Cardio

Wall Pilates:

Breathing Exercises and Warm-up

Core Basics Positions

Integrated Cardio Fitness:

15 minutes of light jogging or jump rope exercises

Day 2: Cardiovascular Enhancement with Arm Strength

Wall Pilates:

Arm Strengthening Exercises

Continuous Flow of Movement

Integrated Cardio Fitness:

High-intensity circuit with light weightlifting exercises

Day 3: Full-body with Intense Cardio

Wall Pilates:

Full Movement Flow

Base Positions with Emphasis on Legs

Integrated Cardio Fitness:

20 minutes of interval training (sprint and recovery) such as stationary running or mountain climbers

Day 4: Active Recovery and Light Cardio

Wall Pilates:

Relaxation and Breathing Exercises

Dynamic Stretching

Integrated Cardio Fitness:

A brisk walk or light cycling for 20-30 minutes

Day 5: Cardio Power with Core Focus

Wall Pilates:

Shoulder Mobility Exercises

Advanced Core Exercises

Integrated Cardio Fitness:

Circuit training with specific core exercises and light running

Important Note:

Adjust the intensity level for both Pilates and cardio exercises based on your fitness level.

Ensure proper technique for each exercise and monitor your cardiovascular response during the workout.

This integrated program offers an effective combination of Wall Pilates and cardio fitness, providing a variety of stimuli to promote strength, flexibility, and optimal cardiovascular health.

Functional Training in the Context of "Wall Pilates for Women"

In the context of Wall Pilates for women, functional training focuses on integrating movements that enhance the body's functionality in everyday life. The goal is to develop strength, flexibility, and coordination through exercises that mimic the body's natural movements. Here's how functional training fits into this context:

Key Principles:

Natural Movements:

Wall Pilates exercises are adapted to mimic everyday movements, such as bending, lifting, pushing, and pulling. This aims to improve the body's ability to handle common activities.

Whole-Body Engagement:

Functional training in Wall Pilates engages the entire body, including the upper and lower limbs, to improve coordination and strength across all body regions.

Multiplanar Exercises:

Exercises include movements in multiple directions to stimulate different muscle chains and improve stability in real-life situations.

Stability and Balance:

Functional training in Wall Pilates places a strong emphasis on core stability and balance, helping to improve posture and reduce the risk of injuries.

Adaptability to Different Abilities:

Functional exercises in the context of Wall Pilates can be adapted for women of different ages and fitness levels, ensuring a personalized approach.

Integration with Pilates Principles:

Functional training is integrated with the fundamental principles of Pilates, such as control, precision, and breathing, creating synergy between the two approaches.

Application in Everyday Life:

The goal is to translate the skills acquired through functional training in Wall Pilates into tangible improvements in daily life.

Functional training in the context of Wall Pilates for women aims to enhance movement quality, functional strength, and the ability to tackle everyday challenges, creating a direct link between training and daily life.

Functional Workouts Integrated with Wall Pilates for Women

Exercise: Wall Ball Squats

Place a fitness ball between your back and the wall.

Perform squats while keeping your back against the ball.

Integrate Wall Pilates movements like raised arms or abdominal contractions.

Exercise: Dynamic Wall Plank with Wall Push-ups

Start in a plank position with your hands against the wall.

Perform elbow push-ups, pushing your body back towards the wall.

Integrate Pilates exercises such as core contraction during the movement.

Exercise: Lateral Lunges with Wall Resistance

Hold a resistance band between your hands, with your body sideways to the wall.

Perform lateral lunges while keeping the band taut.

Integrate Pilates exercises like trunk rotations or side leg lifts.

Exercise: Supine Abdominals with Wall Ball

Place a fitness ball between your feet and lie on your back against the wall.

Perform abdominal exercises by lifting your legs and the ball towards the ceiling.

Integrate core control and Pilates breathing techniques.

Exercise: Side Plank with Leg Lifts

Rest your elbow and forearm against the wall in a side plank position.

Perform side planks with leg lifts.

Integrate Pilates exercises such as abdominal contractions and controlled breathing.

Exercise: Wall-Assisted Tricep Dips with Ball

Position a ball between your back and the wall.

Perform tricep dips while keeping your back against the ball.

Integrate Pilates exercises like abdominal contractions during the movement.

These examples combine functional movements with Wall Pilates principles, offering a comprehensive approach that engages various muscle groups and promotes strength, flexibility, and body control.

Dance in the Context of "Wall Pilates for Women"

In the context of "Wall Pilates for Women," the element of dance is integrated to add an artistic and fluid touch to the exercises. This fusion of Wall Pilates and dance elements aims to promote mind-body connection through graceful and coordinated movements. Here's how the topic of dance fits into this context:

Key Principles:

Creative Expression:

Adding dance elements to Wall Pilates allows women to express their creativity through freer and more fluid movements.

Continuous Flow:

Wall Pilates exercises are performed with a more continuous and harmonious flow, similar to dance choreography, to enhance the fluidity of movement.

Mind-Body Connection:

Dance emphasizes the connection between the mind and body, encouraging a deeper awareness of movement and breathing during exercise.

Enhancement of Flexibility:

Dance elements integrated into Wall Pilates contribute to improving flexibility, allowing for more extensive and controlled movements.

Artistic Exercises:

Some exercises can be structured to incorporate dance-like movements, such as arabesque, plié, and port de bras, adding an artistic aspect to the practice.

Balance and Coordination:

Dance requires a high level of balance and coordination, elements that integrate well with the goals of Wall Pilates.

Variety of Styles:

Dance can be incorporated into various styles, such as ballet, modern, or contemporary, offering a variety of artistic approaches.

Emotional Well-being:

Dance in the context of Wall Pilates can contribute to emotional well-being by providing an opportunity to express emotions through movement.

The integration of dance into Wall Pilates for women offers a creative and artistic approach to training, promoting not only physical strength but also individual expression and emotional well-being.

Pilates on Equipment in the Context of "Wall Pilates for Women"

In the context of "Wall Pilates for Women," the topic of equipment begins by exploring the traditional aspect of Pilates, often involving specialized apparatus. However, the primary focus remains on adapting these principles to the practical and accessible setting of Wall Pilates.

Key Elements of the Topic:

Traditional Pilates Equipment:

Traditional equipment includes the Reformer, Cadillac, Chair, and Barrel. These provide variable resistance to enhance strength and flexibility.

Adaptations to the Wall:

In the context of Wall Pilates for Women, traditional Pilates exercises and principles are adapted for use with the wall as the main support. For example, typical Reformer exercises can be mimicked using the wall for resistance.

Flexibility and Simplicity:

The approach to Wall Pilates maintains a focus on flexibility and simplicity. Using the wall makes exercises accessible to all women without the need for specialized equipment.

Utilizing Vertical Structure:

The wall becomes an ideal partner to leverage the vertical structure. It can be used for stretching exercises, resistance, and to support the body during control and precision exercises.

Concentration on Key Principles:

Even without direct use of traditional apparatus, Wall Pilates maintains a concentration on key principles such as control, breathing, precision, and movement awareness.

Accessibility and Adaptability:

Pilates on Equipment is often considered more advanced, while Wall Pilates for Women focuses on accessibility, adapting exercises to various needs and fitness levels.

In summary, the discussion of equipment in the context of "Wall Pilates for Women" emphasizes the creative adaptation of traditional Pilates principles using the wall as the primary tool, making this practice more accessible and feasible in any home environment.

Relaxation Techniques

In the context of Wall Pilates, relaxation techniques are crucial to enhance body awareness, reduce muscle tension, and improve the quality of movement. Here are some specific relaxation techniques that can be adopted:

Deep Breathing:

Practice diaphragmatic breathing, inhaling slowly through the nose, filling the diaphragm, and then exhaling completely through the mouth. This technique promotes relaxation and breath awareness.

Progressive Muscle Relaxation:

Focus on different parts of the body, briefly contract the muscles, and then completely relax them. Start from the toes and gradually work upward to the head. This helps release muscle tension.

Gentle Stretching:

Integrate gentle and controlled stretching during Wall Pilates. Stretching exercises help release accumulated muscle tension.

Mindful Rest Positions:

Adopt rest positions between exercises, such as Child's Pose, to allow the body to relax and recover. Maintain steady breathing during these pauses.

Mindful Body Awareness:

Practice mindful body awareness during exercises, focusing on sensations and movement. This helps maintain a mind-body connection and reduces stress.

Light Wall-Supported Stretching:

Utilize the wall as support for gentle stretching exercises. For example, lie on the floor with your legs resting vertically against the wall for a relaxing position.

Positive Visualization:

While performing exercises, visualize muscle relaxation and flexibility. Positive visualizations can contribute to reducing mental tension.

Integrating these techniques into your Wall Pilates workout can enhance your overall experience, promote relaxation, and contribute to the overall well-being of both mind and body.

In the end, "Wall Pilates for Women" is more than just an exercise manual; it's a guide that celebrates the strength, flexibility, and empowerment of women through the art of Pilates. Navigating through these pages, you have embarked on a journey of self-discovery, experiencing the transformative power of Wall Pilates.

In this journey, you have learned the fundamentals of Pilates, embracing the principles of control, concentration, precision, fluidity of movement, and breath. You have understood how the wall can become your workout companion, a support that amplifies your practice and connects you deeply with your body.

Through Wall Pilates workouts, you have experienced the restorative ritual of mindful breathing, felt the gentle release of muscle tension, and embraced the grace of controlled movement. The wall has softened your physical and mental boundaries, opening up new possibilities for strength and flexibility.

In your practice, you have learned that Wall Pilates is more than a series of physical exercises. It's an act of kindness towards your body, a dialogue with your mind, and a loving embrace of your authentic self. You have learned that progress is a personal journey, and every step forward is a victory, a reason to celebrate your resilience and commitment.

This book has guided you through specific workouts, providing weekly plans, targeted exercises for beginners and advanced practitioners, and strategies to integrate Wall Pilates into your daily life. You have learned to adapt the practice to your unique needs, celebrate your successes, and face challenges with determination.

But more importantly, you have gained a powerful tool for overall well-being. Wall Pilates goes beyond sculpting the body; it extends to your mental health, awareness, and spiritual connection with yourself. Through Pilates, you have learned that you are stronger than you thought, more flexible than you imagined, and capable of transforming your life.

Looking ahead, remember that Wall Pilates is a constant ally in your pursuit of a healthy and balanced life. Whether you are a beginner learning the basics or an expert refining your practice, the wall will always be there to support you, guide you, and inspire you to surpass your limits.

Be proud of the journey you have undertaken so far, and embrace the path that lies ahead. Whether you are at the wall or away from it, be mindful of your inner strength, nurture your mental flexibility, and continue to breathe with intention. Wall Pilates is a gift you have given yourself, an investment in your health and well-being. Seize this gift and continue to grow, thrive, and shine as the extraordinary woman you are.